WORKBOOK TO ACCOMPANY

FUNDAMENTAL PHARMACOLOGY

For Pharmacy Technicians

Jahangir Moini, MD, MPH, CPhT
Professor and Former Director
Allied Health Sciences, including the Pharmacy Technician Program
Everest University
Melbourne, Florida

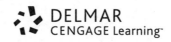

DELMAR
CENGAGE Learning™

Australia • Brazil • Japan • Korea • Mexico • Singapore • Spain • United Kingdom • United States

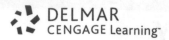

Workbook to accompany Fundamental Pharmacology for Pharmacy Technicians
Jahangir Moini

Vice President, Career and Professional
   Editorial: Dave Garza

Director of Learning Solutions: Matthew Kane

Acquisitions Editor: Tari Broderick

Managing Editor: Marah Bellegarde

Senior Product Manager: Darcy M. Scelsi

Editorial Assistant: Anthony Souza

Vice President, Career and Professional
   Marketing: Jennifer Baker

Marketing Manager: Kristin McNary

Marketing Coordinator: Erika Ropitsky

Production Director: Carolyn Miller

Production Manager: Andrew Crouth

Content Project Manager: Katie Wachtl

Senior Art Director: Jack Pendleton

Library of Congress Control Number: 2009927153

ISBN-13: 978-1-4390-5586-1

ISBN-10: 1-4390-5586-6

Delmar
Executive Woods
5 Maxwell Drive
Clifton Park, NY 12065
USA

Cengage Learning is a leading provider of customized learning solutions with office locations around the globe, including Singapore, the United Kingdom, Australia, Mexico, Brazil, and Japan. Locate your local office at **www.cengage.com/global**

Cengage Learning products are represented in Canada by Nelson Education, Ltd.

To learn more about Delmar, visit **www.cengage.com/delmar**

Purchase any of our products at your local bookstore or at our preferred online store **www.cengagebrain.com**

Notice to the Reader
Publisher does not warrant or guarantee any of the products described herein or perform any independent analysis in connection with any of the product information contained herein. Publisher does not assume, and expressly disclaims, any obligation to obtain and include information other than that provided to it by the manufacturer. The reader is expressly warned to consider and adopt all safety precautions that might be indicated by the activities described herein and to avoid all potential hazards. By following the instructions contained herein, the reader willingly assumes all risks in connection with such instructions. The publisher makes no representations or warranties of any kind, including but not limited to, the warranties of fitness for particular purpose or merchantability, nor are any such representations implied with respect to the material set forth herein, and the publisher takes no responsibility with respect to such material. The publisher shall not be liable for any special, consequential, or exemplary damages resulting, in whole or part, from the readers' use of, or reliance upon, this material.

Printed in the United States of America
2 3 4 5 6   19 18 17 16 15

TABLE OF CONTENTS

General Aspects of Pharmacology

CHAPTER 1

Introduction to Pharmacology, Drug Legislation, and Regulation

Multiple Choice

Select the correct answer from choices A–D.

1. In which of the following periods of pharmacological developments did morphine first begin to be used?

   A. the age of natural substances
   B. the age of biotechnology
   C. the age of synthetic substances
   D. the Middle Ages

2. A human gene can be inserted into one fungal cell. This process is referred to as:

   A. recombinant DNA and RNA technology
   B. recombinant RNA technology
   C. recombinant DNA technology
   D. all of the above

3. In the United States, the development of new drugs can take as long as how many years?

   A. 3
   B. 5
   C. 10
   D. 15

4. Which of the following organizations oversees the approval of new drugs?

   A. CDC
   B. DEA
   C. FDA
   D. The Joint Commission

5. Which of the following stages of drug product development can determine the safety and effectiveness of the drug on animal pharmacology?

   A. Stage 1
   B. Stage 2
   C. Stage 3
   D. Stage 4

6. Which of the following acts requires manufacturers to be concerned with the strength, effectiveness, safety, and packaging of drugs?

   A. the Harrison Narcotic Act of 1914
   B. the Comprehensive Drug Abuse Prevention and Control Act of 1970
   C. the Pure Food, Drug, and Cosmetic Act of 1938
   D. the Pure Food and Drug Act of 1906

7. Tylenol with codeine is listed in Schedule:

   A. I
   B. II
   C. III
   D. IV

8. Cough syrups with codeine are listed in Schedule:

   A. IV
   B. III
   C. II
   D. I

9. Investigational New Drug Review occurs in which of the following stages of drug approval?

   A. 1
   B. 2
   C. 3
   D. 4

10. Which of the following agencies has the authority to designate prescription drugs?

    A. DEA
    B. FDA
    C. DHHS
    D. the Joint Commission

Matching—Drugs and Uses

Match the lettered drug to its numbered description.

Description

1. _____ Low abuse potential; accepted medical use
2. _____ Moderate abuse potential; accepted medical use
3. _____ High abuse potential; no accepted medical use
4. _____ High abuse potential; accepted medical use
5. _____ Low abuse potential; no prescription needed

Drug

A. cough syrups with codeine

B. mescaline

C. diazepam

D. fentanyl

E. acetaminophen with codeine

Fill in the Blank

Select terms from your reading to fill in the blanks.

1. The CSA classifies drugs with the potential for abuse into _____ schedules.

2. The DEA is concerned with controlled substances only, and enforces laws against _____ activities.

3. The FDA is concerned with _____ standards in the production of drugs, food, and cosmetics.

4. The use of natural substances evolved in China and _____.

5. Biotechnology is defined as the use of _____ from cells and tissues from humans, animals, and plants to produce _____ and therapeutic treatments.

6. The _____ is a branch of the U.S. Department of Health and Human Services.

7. Clinical testing on humans takes place in _____ different phases called *clinical phase trials*.

8. Postmarketing surveillance is the _____ stage of the drug approval process.

9. Prescription drugs are also called _____ drugs.

10. The _____ is a part of the U.S. Department of Justice.

11. The Harrison Narcotic Act regulated the importation, manufacture, sale, and use of _____ and _____.

12. The Pure Food, Drug, and Cosmetic Act of 1938 gave the FDA additional control over the _____ and sale of _____.

13. The FDA approves the investigational use of drugs on _____ and ensures that all approved drugs are _____ and _____.

14. The Pure Food and Drug Act was the government's _____ attempt to control and regulate the manufacture, distribution, and _____ of drugs.

15. Schedule V controlled substances have _____ abuse potential and _____ medical use.

True or False

Select the letter "T" or "F" for the following questions.

____ 1. The Pure Food and Drug Act was the government's first attempt to control and regulate the manufacture, distribution, and sale of drugs.

____ 2. The DEA is responsible for the approval and removal from the market of many products.

____ 3. In 1970, the Harrison Narcotic Act was replaced by the Pure Food, Drug, and Cosmetic Act.

____ 4. Schedule III requires prescriptions with only 5 refills permitted in 6 months.

____ 5. Schedule II requires prescriptions with only 2 refills permitted in 6 months.

____ 6. A controlled substance can only legally be obtained with a physician's prescription.

____ 7. Biotechnology is defined as the use of sugars from cells and tissues from humans or plants to produce medicines and therapeutic treatments.

____ 8. In about 2000 B.C., the Chinese began developing an interest in herbs as having value in the cure of disease.

____ 9. Pharmacology is the study of the functions of the body.

____ 10. Drugs that produce a sedative or pain relieving effect are referred to as narcotics.

Matching—Terms and Descriptions

Match the following vocabulary terms and their descriptions.

Terms	Descriptions
1. _____ Genetic engineering	A. Schedules I and II
2. _____ Drug Enforcement Agency	B. Splice genes from one organism into the chromosomes of another organism
3. _____ Pharmacology	C. Human drug testing that is submitted to the FDA once enough data has been collected on a new drug
4. _____ Legend drug	D. Drugs recognized by the DEA as having abuse potential
5. _____ Food and Drug Administration	E. Concerned with controlled substances; enforces laws against illegal drug use
6. _____ Over-the-counter	F. A prescription drug
7. _____ Controlled substances	G. Also known as *recombinant DNA technology*
8. _____ Investigational new drug application	H. The science concerned with drugs and their sources
9. _____ Recombinant DNA	I. Nonprescription drugs technology
10. _____ High abuse potential	J. The branch of the U.S. Department of Health and Human Services which regulates drugs

ANSWER KEY

Multiple Choice

1. A	2. C	3. D	4. C	5. A
6. C	7. C	8. A	9. C	10. B

Matching—Drugs and Uses

1. C	2. E	3. B	4. D	5. A

Fill in the Blank

1. five	2. drug	3. general safety
4. Egypt	5. proteins; medicines	6. FDA
7. three	8. fourth	9. legend
10. DEA	11. opium; codeine	12. manufacture; cosmetics
13. humans; safe; effective	14. first; sale	15. low; accepted

True or False

1. T	2. F	3. F	4. T	5. F
6. T	7. F	8. T	9. F	10. T

Matching—Terms and Descriptions

1. J	2. I	3. H	4. G	5. B
6. D	7. A	8. C	9. F	10. E

CHAPTER 2

Drug Sources and Dosage Forms

Multiple Choice

Select the correct answer from choices A–D.

1. The nonproprietary name is often referred to as the:

   A. generic name
   B. chemical name

   C. trade name
   D. non-chemical name

2. Atropine sulfate and nicotine are examples of:

   A. physical properties
   B. chemical compounds

   C. mineral products
   D. synthetic substances

3. Digoxin is made from:

   A. plants
   B. animals

   C. minerals
   D. engineered drugs

4. Which of the following drug sources is used to prevent severe rheumatoid arthritis?

   A. silver
   B. iron

   C. potassium
   D. gold

5. Which of the following is an example of a synthetic drug?

   A. digoxin
   B. insulin

   C. meperidine
   D. morphine sulfate

6. A pharmaceutical preparation made by compressing the powdered form of a drug under high pressure is called a:

   A. capsule
   B. granule

   C. tablet
   D. plaster

7. Which of the following medications is used to remove corns?

   A. salicylic acid plaster
   B. potassium chloride powder

   C. zinc oxide ointment
   D. nitroglycerin patch

8. Which of the following is an example of a solution?

   A. ipecac fluid
   B. normal saline

   C. iodine tincture
   D. glycyrrhiza fluidextract

7

9. Which of the following gases is used as an anesthetic agent?

   A. carbon dioxide
   B. nitrous oxide

   C. nitrogen mustard
   D. carbon monoxide

10. A small, solid body shaped for ready introduction into one of the orifices of the body is called a:

    A. pill
    B. lozenge

    C. granule
    D. suppository

Matching—Drugs and Descriptions

Match the lettered drug to its numbered description.

Description	Drug
1. _____ A liquid dosage form that contains solid drug particles floating in a liquid	A. Mixture
2. _____ A very small pill, usually gelatin- or sugar-coated, containing a drug to be given in a small dose	B. Spirit
3. _____ A solid preparation that can be spread when heated, and then becomes adhesive at the temperature of the body	C. Suppository
4. _____ An alcoholic solution prepared from vegetable materials, used as a skin disinfectant	D. Plaster
5. _____ Alcoholic or hydroalcoholic solutions of volatile substances	E. Liniment
6. _____ Is solid at ordinary temperatures but melts at body temperature	F. Granule
7. _____ A mutual incorporation of two or more substances, without chemical union, in which the physical characteristics of each of the components are retained	G. Tincture
8. _____ A liquid preparation for external use, usually applied by friction to the skin	H. Suspension

Fill in the Blank

Select terms from your reading to fill in the blanks.

1. A trade name is developed by the _____.

2. Any drug may have dozens of _____ names or trade names.

3. Chemical names and generic names are unique to each _____.

4. Sodium chloride (table salt) is one of the best-known examples of _____ sources.

5. Drug dosage forms are classified according to their physical state and _____ composition.

6. Tablets, powders, and plasters are examples of _____ drugs.

7. A single-dose unit of medicine made by mixing the powdered drug with a liquid is called a _____.

8. An oil-based medication that is enclosed in a soft gelatin capsule is referred to as a _____.

9. A semisolid preparation that is usually white and nongreasy, with a water base, is known as a _____.

10. Liquid drugs are very popular for use in _____ because other oral forms, such as tablets, are harder to swallow.

True or False

Select the letter "T" or "F" for the following questions.

____ 1. An oil-based medication that is enclosed in a soft gelatin capsule is called a gel.

____ 2. A liniment is a liquid preparation for external use, usually applied by friction to the skin.

____ 3. A troche is also called a "lozenge."

____ 4. A drug vehicle that consist of water and sugar is known as an elixir.

____ 5. A drug dosage form that consists of a low concentration of a sugar in water is called a syrup.

____ 6. Most creams and lotions are emulsions.

____ 7. Fluidextracts are not intended to be administered directly to a patient.

____ 8. Chemical names and generic names are unique to each drug.

____ 9. Certain drugs are soluble in water, some are soluble in alcohol, and others are insoluble in a mixture of liquids.

____ 10. Chewable tablets are commonly used for the treatment of asthma and angina pectoris.

ANSWER KEY

Multiple Choice

1. A	2. B	3. A	4. D	5. C
6. C	7. A	8. B	9. B	10. D

Matching—Drugs and Descriptions

1. H	2. F	3. D	4. G
5. B	6. C	7. A	8. E

Fill in the Blank

1. manufacturer	2. brand	3. drug	4. mineral
5. chemical	6. solid	7. pill	8. gelcap
9. cream	10. children		

True or False

1. F	2. T	3. T	4. F	5. F
6. T	7. T	8. T	9. F	10. F

CHAPTER 3

Biopharmaceutics

Multiple Choice

Select the correct answer from choices A–D.

1. The movement of water and dissolved substances from the glomerulus to the Bowman's capsule is referred to as:

   A. excretion
   B. absorption

   C. filtration
   D. biotransformation

2. The most common and important mode of transversal of drugs through membranes is diffusion or:

   A. passive transport
   B. active transport

   C. osmosis
   D. none of the above

3. Which of the following terms indicates measurement of both the rate of drug absorption and total amount of drug that reaches the systemic blood circulation from an administered dosage form?

   A. dose-effect relationship
   B. pharmacodynamic

   C. biotransformation
   D. bioavailability

4. Which of the following organs of the body is the major site of biotransformation?

   A. kidney
   B. liver

   C. lung
   D. small intestine

5. Probenecid may be used to block the renal excretion of which of the following agents?

   A. uric acid
   B. heparin

   C. propranolol
   D. penicillin

6. Which of the following drugs are affected by diurnal body rhythms?

   A. sedatives
   B. analgesics

   C. antacids
   D. antiemetics

7. *Pharmacodynamics* means:

   A. the study of drugs derived from herbal and other natural sources
   B. the study of the biochemical and physiological effects of drugs

   C. the study of drugs, including their actions and side effects
   D. the study of the biotransformation of drugs

8. The rate of filtration in the glomerulus is normally _____ milliliters per minute.

   A. 65
   B. 95

   C. 125
   D. 175

9. Which of the following substances can convert most drugs to their metabolic derivatives during metabolism?

   A. vitamins
   B. enzymes

   C. hormones
   D. none of the above

10. Hepatic portal circulation carries blood directly to the:

    A. stomach
    B. lung

    C. heart
    D. liver

11. Active transport is the process that moves particles in fluid through membranes from:

    A. a region of higher concentration to a region of lower concentration
    B. a region of lower concentration to a region of higher concentration

    C. an extracellular to an intracellular region
    D. none of the above

12. Which of the following factors may influence intensity of drug effects?

    A. drug allergy
    B. drug price

    C. tolerance
    D. metabolism

13. Cell membranes consist of a fatty bi-layer through which drugs must pass for _____ to occur.

    A. drug elimination
    B. drug reabsorption

    C. drug filtration
    D. diffusion

14. A drug that blocks a functional change in the cell is known as:

    A. a bioavailable drug
    B. an antagonist

    C. an agonist
    D. a bio-transformed drug

15. The majority of drug metabolites are:

    A. useful and beneficial
    B. active and nontoxic
    C. inactive and toxic

    D. known to increase the life spans of red blood cells

16. Tubular secretion involves the active secretion of substances such as potassium (K^+) ions, hydrogen (H^+) ions, uric acid, and which of the following substances?

    A. sodium ions and drugs
    B. ammonium ions and drugs

    C. red blood cells and drugs
    D. all of the above

17. The *first-pass effect* means:

    A. that drugs reach the liver, where they are partially metabolized before being sent to the body
    B. that drugs reach the liver, where they are completely metabolized before being sent to the body

    C. that drugs reach the blood circulation from the small intestine
    D. none of the above

18. A sugar pill is an example of a:

    A. pain killer
    B. neurotoxin

    C. phytotoxin
    D. placebo

19. A substance that is produced to alter the actions of liver enzymes is referred to as:

    A. a plasma protein
    B. an antimetabolite

    C. an antagonist
    D. an agonist

20. The term "half-life" describes which of the following?

    A. The time it takes for the plasma concentration to be increased by 50 percent
    B. The time it takes for the plasma concentration to be increased by 90 percent

    C. The time it takes for the plasma concentration to be reduced by 50 percent
    D. The time it takes for the plasma concentration to be reduced by 90 percent

Matching—Terms and Descriptions

Match the lettered term to its numbered description.

1. _____ A process that moves particles in fluid through membranes from a region of lower concentration to a region of higher concentration

2. _____ The study of the action and movement of drugs within the body

3. _____ The study of the biochemical and physiological effects of drugs

4. _____ The conversion of a drug within the body

5. _____ Reduced responsiveness of a drug because of adaptation to it

A. Tolerance

B. Metabolism

C. Pharmacokinetic

D. Pharmacodynamic

E. Active transport

Matching—Drugs and Responses

Match the lettered drug response to its numbered description.

1. _____ Usually imply more severe symptoms or problems that develop because of a drug

2. _____ Severe allergic reactions that are life-threatening

3. _____ Referred to as *mild responses to a drug*

4. _____ Unique, strange, or unpredicted reactions to a drug

5. _____ Hypersensitivity reactions that some drugs may cause in certain patients

A. Idiosyncratic reactions

B. Anaphylactic reactions

C. Allergies

D. Side effects

E. Adverse effects

Fill in the Blank

Select terms from your reading to fill in the blanks.

1. Agents that are relatively lipid-soluble diffuse _____ than less lipid-soluble drugs.

2. For absorption to occur, a drug must be transported across biological _____ to reach the blood circulation.

3. Oral administration of drugs is the most _____, economical, and _____ route of administration.

4. Drugs with an acidic pH are easily _____ in the _____ environment of the stomach.

5. Drugs administered in high concentrations tend to be more _____ absorbed than when administered in low _____.

6. The brain and placenta possess special anatomical _____ that prevent many chemicals and drugs from entering.

7. Liver enzymes react with drugs, creating _____.

8. Alcohol, cocaine, and nicotine easily cross the placental _____ and can potentially _____ the fetus.

9. Patients with liver _____ may require lower dosages of a drug.

10. Unchanged drugs or drug metabolites mostly can be eliminated by the _____.

11. The rate of filtration is referred to as the _____ filtration rate, and is normally 125 to 130 _____ per minute.

12. Secretions of drugs are active transport systems and require _____.

13. Drug clearance describes drug _____.

14. Drug action is generally described relative to a physiological state that was in existence when a drug was _____.

15. Newborns and _____ individuals show the greatest effects of a _____.

True or False

____ 1. The movement of drugs through the body is called "pharmacodynamics."

____ 2. Measurement of the rate of absorption and total amount of drug that reaches the systemic circulation is known as "biotransformation."

____ 3. Filtration causes water and dissolved substances to move from the glomerulus into the Bowman's capsule.

____ 4. Probenecid may be used to block the renal excretion of penicillin.

____ 5. By altering the pH of urine, increased elimination of certain drugs can be facilitated, thus preventing prolonged action or overdosage of a toxic compound.

____ 6. Drug action is generally described relative to a physiological state that was in existence when administered.

____ 7. Drug clearance describes drug absorption.

____ 8. Acute or chronic disorders of the liver in elderly patients may cause severe toxicity.

____ 9. Effects of medications taken together are called "adverse effects."

____ 10. An anaphylactic reaction is not a medical emergency.

ANSWER KEY

Multiple Choice

1. C	2. A	3. D	4. B	5. D
6. A	7. B	8. C	9. B	10. C
11. B	12. D	13. D	14. B	15. C
16. B	17. A	18. D	19. B	20. C

Matching—Terms and Descriptions

1. E	2. C	3. D	4. B	5. A

Matching—Drugs and Responses

1. E	2. B	3. D	4. A	5. C

Fill in the Blank

1. more rapidly	2. membranes	3. convenient; common
4. absorbed; acid	5. rapidly; concentration	6. barriers
7. metabolites	8. barrier; harm	9. disease
10. kidneys	11. glomerular; milliliters	12. energy
13. elimination	14. administered	15. elderly; drug's actions

True or False

1. F	2. F	3. T	4. T	5. T
6. T	7. F	8. T	9. F	10. F

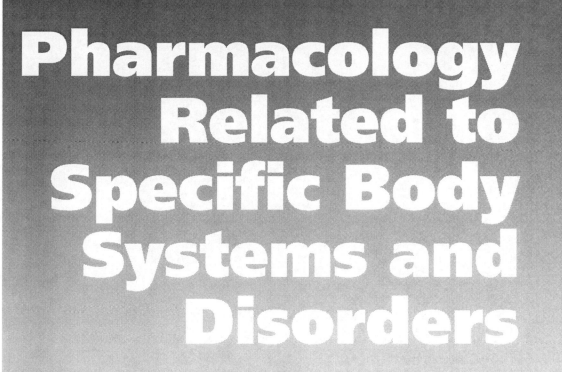

Pharmacology Related to Specific Body Systems and Disorders

CHAPTER 4

Drug Therapy for the Nervous System: Antipsychotic and Antidepressant Drugs

Multiple Choice

Select the correct answer from choices A–D.

1. Which of the following neurotransmitters plays a major role in cognitive function and memory formation, as well as motor control?

   A. gamma-aminobutyric acid
   B. noradrenaline
   C. serotonin
   D. acetylcholine

2. Antipsychotic drugs are also known as:

   A. neurotransmitters
   B. neuroleptics
   C. antidepressants
   D. selective serotonin reuptake inhibitors

3. Which of the following parts of the brain regulates appetite, temperature, fluid levels, hormone production, and biological rhythms?

   A. cerebrum
   B. diencephalon
   C. brainstem
   D. cerebellum

4. Cranial nerves consist of how many pairs?

   A. 2
   B. 5
   C. 12
   D. 26

5. Which of the following disorders can result in alterations in dopamine production?

   A. Parkinson's disease
   B. schizophrenia
   C. attention deficit disorder
   D. all of the above

6. Serotonin is a neurotransmitter synthesized in the central nervous system, as well as:

   A. the gastrointestinal tract
   B. the urinary system
   C. the respiratory system
   D. all of the above

7. Antidepressant effects may not be observed for up to four _____ after treatment begins.

   A. hours
   B. days
   C. weeks
   D. months

8. Which of the following antidepressant drugs may interact with specific foods and cause a hypertensive crisis?

   A. tricyclic antidepressants
   B. monoamine oxidase inhibitors
   C. typical antidepressant drugs
   D. all of the above

9. Which of the following is the trade name of sertraline hydrochloride?

   A. Zoloft®
   B. Paxil®
   C. Prozac®
   D. Tofranil®

10. Tricyclic antidepressants inhibit the reuptake of:

    A. serotonin and acetylcholine
    B. serotonin and noradrenaline
    C. serotonin and dopamine
    D. serotonin and gamma-aminobutyric acid

11. Which of the following agents may be used for the treatment of nighttime bed wetting in children?

    A. paroxetine (Paxil®)
    B. sertraline (Zoloft®)
    C. imipramine (Tofranil®)
    D. nortriptyline (Aventyl®)

12. Spinal nerves consist of how many pairs?

    A. 7
    B. 12
    C. 26
    D. 31

13. Tricyclic antidepressants are contraindicated in patients with all of the following conditions, except:

    A. hypertrophy of the prostate gland
    B. pregnancy or lactation
    C. major depression
    D. glaucoma

14. All of the following are parts of the brain stem, except:

    A. the pons
    B. the hypothalamus
    C. the medulla oblongata
    D. the midbrain

15. Which of the following agents are now considered the first-line drugs in the treatment of major depression?

    A. lithium
    B. TCAs
    C. MAOIs
    D. SSRIs

16. Dementia may occur at any age and can affect young people as the result of injury or:

    A. hypoxia
    B. hypocalcemia
    C. hypokalemia
    D. hyponatremia

17. Schizophrenia is the primary indication for:

    A. mood-altering drugs
    B. antidepressants
    C. antipsychotic drugs
    D. all of the above

18. Which of the following is the generic name of Moban®?

    A. molindone
    B. maprotiline
    C. paroxetine
    D. pimozide

19. SSRIs are used in major depression and may be prescribed for obsessive-compulsive disorder and:

    A. renal dysfunction
    B. insomnia
    C. nervousness
    D. eating disorders

20. Adverse effects of atypical antidepressants include all of the following, except:

    A. blurred vision
    B. insomnia
    C. loss of appetite
    D. orthostatic hypotension

Matching—Terms and Descriptions

Match the lettered term to its numbered description.

Description	Term
1. _____ Controls blood pressure and respiration	A. Cerebrum
2. _____ Controls endocrine system processes, appetite, and sleep	B. Cerebellum
3. _____ Basic functional unit of the nervous system	C. Brainstem
4. _____ Maintains basic muscle tone and coordinates balance	D. Hypothalamus
5. _____ Provides higher mental function	E. Neuron
6. _____ Receives sensory stimuli, except the sense of smell	F. Thalamus

Matching—Drug Names

Match the generic and trade names.

Generic Name	Trade Name
1. _____ pimozide	A. Ludiomil®
2. _____ loxapine	B. Luvox®
3. _____ fluphenazine	C. Elavil®
4. _____ chlorpromazine	D. Mellaril®
5. _____ maprotiline	E. Thorazine®
6. _____ amitriptyline	F. Orap®
7. _____ thioridazine	G. Prolixin®
8. _____ fluvoxamine	H. Loxitane®

Fill in the Blank

Select terms from your reading to fill in the blanks.

1. Sensory nerves are also called _____ nerves.

2. Neurons consist of a cell body, dendrites, and _____.

3. Disorders in the production and function of neurotransmitters may contribute to _____ illnesses.

4. Noradrenaline is also known as _____.

5. _____ is a neurotransmitter that plays an important role in regulating anger, aggression, body temperature, mood, sleep, vomiting, and sexuality.

6. Serotonin syndrome is also known as serotonin _____.

7. Antipsychotic drugs act by blocking receptors for dopamine, acetylcholine, histamine, and _____.

8. Bipolar disorder was formerly known as _____-depressive illness.

9. Lithium is contraindicated in children younger than _____ years of age.

10. Historically, tricyclic antidepressants have been the _____ choice in the treatment of _____.

11. Selective serotonin-reuptake inhibitors are new _____.

12. Hypertensive crisis (severe hypertension) may occur if ingesting foods containing tyramine while taking _____.

13. Atypical antidepressants are also called _____ agents.

14. The brain consists of _____ parts: the cerebrum, _____, cerebellum, and _____.

15. Axons carry impulses _____ from the cell body of the neuron.

True or False

Select the letter "T" or "F" for the following questions.

____ 1. The cerebellum controls blood pressure and pulse.

____ 2. Diencephalon consists of brainstem and cerebrum.

____ 3. The spinal cord provides a two-way communication system between the brain and body parts outside of the nervous system.

____ 4. Decreased production of dopamine plays a role in bulimia nervosa.

____ 5. Chlorpromazine is used for treating hiccups and lithium is used for managing bipolar disorders.

____ 6. Thorazine is the trade name of clozapine.

____ 7. Antipsychotic agents commonly cause adverse effects related to excessive extrapyramidal activity.

____ 8. Lithium is a drug of choice for controlling Parkinson's disease.

____ 9. Prozac is the trade name of fluoxetine.

____ 10. MAOIs are the drug of choice for major depression.

ANSWER KEY

Multiple Choice

1. D	2. B	3. B	4. C	5. D
6. A	7. C	8. B	9. A	10. B
11. C	12. D	13. C	14. B	15. D
16. A	17. C	18. A	19. D	20. C

Matching—Terms and Descriptions

1. C	2. D	3. E	4. B	5. A
6. F				

Matching—Drug Names

1. F	2. H	3. G	4. E	5. A
6. C	7. D	8. B		

Fill in the Blank

1. afferent	2. axons	3. psychiatric
4. norepinephrine	5. Serotonin	6. toxicity
7. norepinephrine	8. manic	9. twelve
10. first; depression	11. antidepressants	12. MAOIs
13. miscellaneous	14. four; diencephalon; brain stem	15. away

True or False

1. F	2. F	3. T	4. F	5. T
6. F	7. T	8. F	9. T	10. F

CHAPTER 5

Drug Therapy for the Nervous System: Antianxiety and Hypnotic Drugs

Multiple Choice

Select the correct answer from choices A–D.

1. Which of the following is the generic name of Luminal®?

    A. butabarbital
    B. phenobarbital

    C. aprobarbital
    D. amobarbital

2. Benzodiazepine-like drugs act as agonists at the benzodiazepine receptor site on the:

    A. receptors for dopamine
    B. receptors for acetylcholine

    C. receptors for histamine
    D. GABA receptor-chloride channel complex

3. An uncomfortable state that has both psychological and physical components is called:

    A. depression
    B. anxiety

    C. insomnia
    D. bulimia

4. Generalized anxiety disorder may last for:

    A. three weeks or longer
    B. six weeks or longer

    C. three months or longer
    D. six months or longer

5. Which of the following stimulates the brain and may reduce the ability to sleep?

    A. quazepam
    B. diazepam

    C. alcohol
    D. secobarbital

6. Which of the following is the trade name of alprazolam?

    A. Klonopin®
    B. Xanax®

    C. Valium®
    D. Paxipam®

7. Benzodiazepines are useful for the short-term treatment of:

    A. panic disorder
    B. insomnia

    C. generalized anxiety
    D. all of the above

8. Which of the following agents can increase levels of prolactin and reduce levels of testosterone?

    A. ramelteon (Rozerem®)
    B. zaleplon (Sonata®)

    C. atenolol (Tenormin®)
    D. propranolol (Inderal®)

25

9. Phenobarbital and mephobarbital are used for:

A. congenital heart defects
B. pyloric stenosis

C. hypotension
D. congenital hyperbilirubinemia

10. Benzodiazepines should be used cautiously in which of the following patients?

A. teenagers
B. elderly patients

C. middle-aged women
D. all of the above

11. All of the following are distinct advantages of buspirone (BuSpar®), except:

A. it has no abuse potential
B. it has no effect on anxiety

C. it does not cause sedation
D. it does not intensify the effects of CNS depressants

12. Which of the following agents have become very popular as sleep aids?

A. beta blockers
B. antiseizure medications

C. nonbenzodiazepine drugs
D. barbiturates

13. Drugs given to promote sleep are known as:

A. sedatives
B. hypnotics

C. niacins
D. all of the above

14. Which of the following terms means a "slower than normal heart rate"?

A. bradycardia
B. fibrillation

C. flutter
D. tachycardia

15. Anxiety and insomnia are treated primarily with benzodiazepines and:

A. SSRIs
B. MAOIs

C. GABA
D. TCA

Matching—Drug Names

Match the generic and trade names.

Generic Name	Trade Name
1. _____ flurazepam	A. Serax®
2. _____ diazepam	B. Seconal®
3. _____ chlordiazepoxide	C. Restoril®
4. _____ secobarbital	D. Klonopin®
5. _____ oxazepam	E. Librium®
6. _____ quazepam	F. Doral®
7. _____ temazepam	G. Valium®
8. _____ clonazepam	H. Dalmane®

Fill in the Blank

Select terms from your reading to fill in the blanks.

1. Overdosage of benzodiazepines may result in CNS and _____ depression as well as hypotension and _____.

2. The benzodiazepines are categorized as Schedule _____ drugs.

3. The phrase "without muscular coordination" defines the term _____.

4. Benzodiazepine-like drugs, especially zolpidem (Ambien®) and buspirone (BuSpar®) are widely used for _____ disorders and _____.

5. Ramelteon is approved for treating chronic _____.

6. Barbiturates cause tolerance and _____, have high abuse potential, and are subject to multiple drug interactions.

7. Thiopental and other highly lipid-soluble barbiturates are given to induce _____.

8. Buspirone does not enhance the depressant effects of _____, barbiturates, and other general CNS _____.

9. The inability to fall asleep is referred to as _____.

10. A drug administered before an anesthetic is called a _____.

11. Panic attacks have a sudden onset, reaching peak intensity within _____ minutes.

12. According to the *American Journal of Psychiatry*, the incidence of panic disorders in women is _____ to _____ times that seen in men.

13. Social anxiety disorders are one of the most common types of _____ disorders.

14. First-line drugs for generalized anxiety disorders and panic disorders are _____.

15. Onset of panic disorder usually occurs in the late _____ or early _____.

True or False

Select the letter "T" or "F" for the following questions.

_____ 1. Drugs that relieve anxiety are also known as "antipsychotics."

_____ 2. A sudden onset (with peak intensity within ten minutes) of symptoms such as shortness of breath, heart palpitations, chest tightness, and sweating signifies a panic attack.

_____ 3. Sleep disturbances are extremely uncommon in the United States.

_____ 4. Generalized anxiety disorder is a chronic condition characterized by uncontrollable worrying.

_____ 5. Social anxiety disorder is formerly known as photophobia.

_____ 6. Benzodiazepines are the first-line drugs for generalized anxiety and panic disorders.

_____ 7. Alprazolam is the generic name of Serax®.

_____ 8. Adverse effects of benzodiazepines are drowsiness, ataxia, impaired judgment, and dry mouth.

_____ 9. Barbiturates can be used to treat insomnia, seizures, and for general anesthesia.

_____ 10. The manifestation of adverse effects of barbiturates include vomiting, diarrhea, and weight gain.

ANSWER KEY

Multiple Choice

1. B	2. D	3. B	4. D	5. C
6. B	7. D	8. A	9. D	10. B
11. B	12. C	13. B	14. A	15. A

Matching—Drug Names

1. H	2. G	3. E	4. B	5. A
6. F	7. C	8. D		

Fill in the Blank

1. respiratory; coma	2. IV (4)	3. ataxia
4. sleep; anxiety	5. insomnia	6. dependence
7. general anesthesia	8. alcohol; depressants	9. insomnia
10. preanesthetic	11. ten	12. two; three
13. psychiatric	14. benzodiazepines	15. teens; twenties

True or False

1. F	2. T	3. F	4. T	5. F
6. T	7. F	8. T	9. T	10. F

CHAPTER 6

Drug Therapy for the Autonomic Nervous System

Multiple Choice

Select the correct answer from choices A–D.

1. Acetylcholine is the chemical transmitter released by:

   A. all preganglionic neurons of the peripheral nervous system
   B. all sensory neurons of the skeletal muscles
   C. all postganglionic neurons of the sympathetic nervous system
   D. all of the above

2. Dopamine receptors respond to which of the following neurotransmitters found primarily in the central nervous system?

   A. norepinephrine only
   B. epinephrine only
   C. dopamine only
   D. norepinephrine, epinephrine, and dopamine

3. Sympathomimetics are also referred to as:

   A. cholinergics
   B. dopanergics
   C. adrenergic blockers
   D. adrenergics

4. Which of the following is the trade name of salmeterol xinafoate?

   A. Dobutrex®
   B. Serevent®
   C. Alupent®
   D. Metaprel®

5. Adrenergic drugs stimulate which of the following receptor sites?

   A. $beta_1$ and $alpha_1$
   B. $alpha_2$ and $beta_2$
   C. $alpha_1$ and $beta_2$
   D. $alpha_2$ and $beta_1$

6. $Beta_2$-adrenergic receptors in the respiratory system are located in the:

   A. trachea
   B. bronchi
   C. bronchial tubes
   D. alveoli

7. Sympatholytic agents are also called:

   A. cholinergics
   B. cholinergic blockers
   C. adrenergic blockers
   D. adrenergic agonists

8. Adrenergic blockers are used in the treatment of which of the following disorders or conditions?

   A. hypertension
   B. heart failure
   C. glaucoma
   D. all of the above

9. At cholinergic transmission sites, some cholinergic drugs increase the concentration of:

   A. dopamine
   B. norepinephrine
   C. epinephrine
   D. acetylcholine

10. Cholinergic agonist drugs are used most commonly in which of the following?

    A. hypertension
    B. glaucoma
    C. pheochromocytoma
    D. asthma

11. The trade name of tacrine is:

    A. Cognex®
    B. Salagen®
    C. Prostigmin®
    D. Exelon®

12. Cholinergic blockers are also known as:

    A. parasympathomimetics
    B. parasympatholytics
    C. sympathomimetics
    D. dopanergics

13. Parasympatholytics act by selectively blocking all muscarine receptors from which of the following neurotransmitters?

    A. norepinephrine
    B. dopamine
    C. epinephrine
    D. acetylcholine

14. Cholinergic blockers are prescribed to produce:

    A. miosis
    B. mydriasis
    C. intestinal atony
    D. excitement

15. Paralysis of the ciliary muscles of the eye is called:

    A. diplopia
    B. amblyopia
    C. nystagmus
    D. cycloplegia

Matching—Terms and Definitions

Match the lettered term to its numbered description.

1. _____ Stimulates skeletal muscle   A. Parasympathomimetics

2. _____ Known as "adrenergics"   B. Parasympatholytics

3. _____ Referred to as "cholinergics"   C. Sympatholytics

4. _____ Called "adrenergic blockers"   D. Sympathomimetics

5. _____ Called "anticholinergics"   E. Somatic motor system

Matching—Drug Names

Match the generic and trade names.

Generic Name   **Trade Name**

1. _____ nadolol   A. Coreg®

2. _____ prazosin   B. Flomax®

3. _____ propranolol   C. Minipress®

4. _____ tamsulosin   D. Inderal®

5. _____ carvedilol   E. Corgard®

Fill in the Blank

Select terms from your reading to fill in the blanks.

1. Adrenergic blockers reduce delivery of _____.

2. Because the thermal regulatory system in elderly people declines, hyperthermia is possible with _____. This happens because these agents decrease _____.

3. The sympathetic division of the peripheral nervous system controls the response known as "_____."

4. The parasympathetic division of the peripheral nervous system controls the response known as "_____."

5. The somatic motor system releases _____ and stimulates _____ muscle.

6. All autonomic nervous system ganglia, and the adrenal medulla, contain the _____ receptor subtype.

7. Adrenergic drugs stimulate both alpha$_1$ and _____ receptor sites.

8. Beta-adrenergic drugs are used in the treatment of respiratory conditions such as _____ and _____.

9. The trade name of acebutolol is _____.

10. A drug that acts to oppose the actions of the sympathetic nervous system is referred to as _____.

11. Pheochromocytoma is a pigmented tumor of the chromaffin cells of the _____ gland.

12. Some cholinergic drugs increase the concentration of _____ at cholinergic transmission sites, which prolongs and exaggerates their action.

13. The routes of administration of neostigmine (Prostigmin®) include PO, _____, and _____.

14. Cholinergic agonist drugs are used most commonly for glaucoma by inducing _____.

15. Congenital megacolon is due to reduction in motor neurons of the _____ nervous system and results in extreme constipation.

16. Some cholinergic drugs increase concentration of acetylcholine at cholinergic transmission sites, which _____ and _____ their action.

17. Inflammation of the vascular middle layer of the eye, including the iris, ciliary body, and choroid, is called _____.

18. Postganglionic terminal axons of the sympathetic nervous system in sweat glands releases _____.

19. The route of administration of salmeterol (Serevent®) is _____.

20. The route of administration for oxymetazoline (Afrin®) is _____.

True or False

Select the letter "T" or "F" for the following questions.

____ 1. A catecholamine is one of a group of chemically related compounds having a sympathomimetic action.

____ 2. Somnolence is defined as prolonged drowsiness that may last hours to days.

____ 3. Dilation of the pupils of the eyes is called *miosis*.

____ 4. Epinephrine is a major transmitter released by the adrenal cortex.

____ 5. Muscarinic receptors are located in all parasympathetic target organs of the body systems.

____ 6. Adrenergic agonist drugs may affect both alpha- and beta-receptors.

____ 7. Ventolin® is the trade name of methyldopa.

____ 8. Adrenergic drugs stimulate only alpha$_2$ receptor sites.

____ 9. No clinically significant drug interactions have been established for alpha-adrenergic agents.

____ 10. Regitine® and Cartrol® are the trade names of nadolol and propranolol.

ANSWER KEY

Multiple Choice

1. A	2. C	3. D	4. B	5. C
6. C	7. C	8. D	9. D	10. B
11. A	12. B	13. D	14. B	15. D

Matching—Terms and Definitions

1. E	2. D	3. A	4. C	5. B

Matching—Drug Names

1. E	2. C	3. D	4. B	5. A

Fill in the Blank

1. catecholamines
2. anticholinergics; sweating
3. Fight or Flight
4. Rest or Digest
5. acetylcholine; skeletal
6. nicotinic-$_N$
7. beta$_2$
8. asthma; bronchitis
9. Sectral®
10. sympatholytic
11. adrenal
12. acetylcholine
13. IM; IV
14. miosis
15. parasympathetic
16. prolongs; exaggerates
17. uveitis
18. acetylcholine
19. inhalation
20. intranasal

True or False

1. T	2. T	3. F	4. F	5. T
6. T	7. F	8. F	9. T	10. F

CHAPTER 7

Drug Therapy for Parkinson's and Alzheimer's Diseases

Multiple Choice

Select the correct answer from choices A–D.

1. Parkinson's disease causes dysfunction and changes in which of the following parts of the brain?

   A. pons
   B. cerebellum

   C. basal nuclei
   D. brain stem

2. Parkinson's disease usually develops after age:

   A. 40
   B. 50

   C. 60
   D. 80

3. Anti-parkinsonism drugs are administered to restore the balance of:

   A. dopamine and acetylcholine
   B. dopamine and epinephrine

   C. dopamine and serotonin
   D. norepinephrine and acetylcholine

4. All of the following agents may be prescribed for a patient with parkinsonism, except:

   A. tacrine (Cognex®)
   B. levodopa (Larodopa®)

   C. bromocriptine (Parlodel®)
   D. amantadine (Symmetrel®)

5. Acetylcholinesterase inhibitors slow the neuronal degradation that occurs in which of the following?

   A. Parkinson's disease
   B. Alzheimer's disease

   C. absence seizure
   D. panic attacks

6. Levodopa should be avoided in patients with all of the following conditions, except:

   A. receiving an MAO inhibitor
   B. during lactation

   C. parkinsonism
   D. narrow-angle glaucoma

7. Ginkgo is a natural remedy, and is used in treating which of the following conditions?

   A. dementia
   B. seizures

   C. anemia
   D. inability to sleep

8. Patients taking levodopa should be monitored for:

   A. fever
   B. loss of vision

   C. orthostatic hypotension
   D. increase in the number of white blood cells

9. Which of the following is the most common cause of severe cognitive dysfunction in older patients?

    A. bipolar disorder   C. bulimia nervosa
    B. anorexia nervosa   D. Alzheimer's disease

10. The trade name of donepezil is:

    A. Razadyne®   C. Exelon®
    B. Aricept®   D. Cognex®

11. Alzheimer's disease is a devastating illness characterized by all of the following, except:

    A. disorientation   C. muscular rigidity
    B. impaired thinking   D. memory failure

12. A decrease in spontaneity and movement, as seen in Parkinson's disease, is referred to as:

    A. bradykinesia   C. bradyarrhythmia
    B. bradycardia   D. hyperthermia

13. Which of the following neurotransmitter imbalances is exhibited in Parkinson's disease?

    A. high dopamine and low acetylcholine   C. high acetylcholine and high dopamine
    B. high acetylcholine and high norepinephrine   D. high acetylcholine and low dopamine

14. Which of the following is a significant risk from using tacrine (Cognex®)?

    A. liver damage   C. hypertension
    B. darkened stool   D. hair loss

15. Kemadrin® is the trade name of:

    A. biperiden   C. procyclidine
    B. diphenhydramine   D. none of the above

Matching—Drug Names

Match the generic and trade names.

Generic Name	Trade Name
1. _____ procyclidine	A. Symmetrel®
2. _____ biperiden	B. Carbex®
3. _____ amantadine	C. Permax®
4. _____ selegiline	D. Akineton®
5. _____ pergolide	E. Kemadrin®

Matching—Terms and Descriptions

Match the following vocabulary terms and their descriptions.

1. _____ Atrophy	A.	Repetitive movements, but irregular contraction of opposing muscle groups
2. _____ Substantia nigra	B.	A layer of nervous tissue within the brain
3. _____ Corpus striatum	C.	Clusters of nerve cells at the base of the brain; responsible for body movement and coordination
4. _____ Basal nuclei	D.	Pigmented cells in the midbrain responsible for the production of dopamine
5. _____ Tremor	E.	Wasting away, or "without development"

Fill in the Blank

Select terms from your reading to fill in the blanks.

1. It is estimated that as many as _____ Americans have Parkinson's disease.

2. The cause of Parkinson's disease is _____.

3. Encephalitis means _____ of the brain.

4. Anti-parkinsonism drugs are administered to restore the balance of _____ and acetylcholine.

5. Levodopa is a precursor of _____ formation and stimulates the process of balance needed to treat Parkinson's disease.

6. Parkinson's disease is characterized by a _____ gait and early postural changes.

7. Patients with Alzheimer's disease should receive pharmacotherapy for at least _____ months prior to assessing the maximum _____ of drug therapy.

8. Hepatotoxicity means _____ poisoning.

9. Hallucinations occur commonly in older adults when taking _____ receptor agonists.

10. Levodopa is considered the drug of choice for _____ disease.

11. Parkinson's disease may occur following _____, _____, or vascular disease.

12. Dopaminergic drugs affect _____.

13. Amantadine is less effective than levodopa as a drug therapy for _____ disease.

14. Amantadine is also indicated for drug therapy for _____ disorders.

15. Cholinergic blockers are used as adjunctive therapy to relieve _____ symptoms.

True or False

Select the letter "T" or "F" for the following questions.

____ 1. Patients taking levodopa can have foods containing substantial amounts of pyridoxine (vitamin B_6)

____ 2. The exact cause of Alzheimer's disease is unknown.

____ 3. Alzheimer's disease is also called senile disease complex.

____ 4. *Leukopenia* means a decrease in red blood cells.

____ 5. In Alzheimer's disease, acetylcholine is increased.

____ 6. Acetylcholinesterase inhibitors are used in the treatment of mild to moderate dementia of the Alzheimer's type.

____ 7. Donepezil and tacrine increase effects and risks of toxicity with theophylline.

____ 8. Acetylcholinesterase inhibitors should be used cautiously in patients with cardiac disorders.

____ 9. Donepezil may cause darkened urine.

____ 10. The FDA has approved numerous medications for Alzheimer's disease.

ANSWER KEY

Multiple Choice

1. C	2. C	3. A	4. A	5. B
6. C	7. A	8. C	9. D	10. B
11. C	12. A	13. D	14. A	15. C

Matching—Drug Names

1. E	2. D	3. A	4. B	5. C

Matching—Terms and Descriptions

1. E	2. D	3. B	4. C	5. A

Fill in the Blank

1. 1.5 million	2. unknown	3. inflammation
4. dopamine	5. dopamine	6. shuffling
7. six; benefits	8. liver	9. dopamine
10. Parkinson's	11. encephalitis; trauma	12. dopamine
13. Parkinson's	14. viral	15. parkinsonism

True or False

1. F	2. T	3. T	4. F	5. F
6. T	7. T	8. T	9. T	10. F

Drug Therapy for Seizures

Multiple Choice

Select the correct answer from choices A–D.

1. Which of the following include partial seizures?

   A. tonic-clonic
   B. petit mal
   C. Jacksonian
   D. atonic

2. Absence seizures are also referred to as which of the following?

   A. akinetic
   B. petit mal
   C. Jacksonian
   D. grand mal

3. The most recognizable and used drug in the hydantoin class is:

   A. felbamate
   B. valproic acid
   C. ethosuximide
   D. phenytoin

4. Which of the following antiseizure drugs is used for the prevention of migraine headaches?

   A. valproic acid (Depakene®)
   B. phenytoin (Dilantin®)
   C. pregabalin (Lyrica®)
   D. zonisamide (Zonegran®)

5. Hydantoin agents are contraindicated in patients with which of the following conditions?

   A. seizures due to low blood glucose
   B. pregnancy and lactation
   C. rash
   D. all of the above

6. Phenytoin-like drugs are contraindicated in patients with which of the following conditions or diseases?

   A. cardiac disorders
   B. renal diseases
   C. pregnancy and lactation
   D. all of the above

7. Which of the following succinimide drugs is considered to be the safest and most commonly prescribed anticonvulsant?

   A. ethosuximide (Zarontin®)
   B. methsuximide (Celontin®)
   C. valproic acid (Depakene®)
   D. felbamate (Felbatol®)

8. Complex seizures are also called:

   A. psychomotor
   B. tonic-clonic
   C. myoclonic
   D. absence

9. Recurrent or continuous seizures without recovery of consciousness are termed:

   A. grand mal seizures
   B. psychomotor seizures
   C. status epilepticus
   D. atonic seizures

10. Luminal® is the trade name of:

   A. propranolol®
   B. clonazepam

   C. diazepam
   D. phenobarbital sodium

11. The indications of benzodiazepines include all of the following, except:

   A. food poisoning
   B. alcohol withdrawal symptoms

   C. skeletal muscle spasms
   D. anxiety

12. Phenytoin is used for all of the following, except:

   A. head trauma
   B. hyperglycemia

   C. psychomotor seizures
   D. tonic-clonic seizures

13. Which of the following phenytoin-like drugs may be used for the treatment of bipolar disorder?

   A. carbamazepine (Tegretol®)
   B. valproic acid (Depakene®)

   C. pregabalin (Lyrica®)
   D. zonisamide (Zonegran®)

14. Succinimide drugs are used to control which of the following seizures?

   A. infantile spasms
   B. tonic-clonic (grand mal)

   C. absence (petit mal)
   D. simple seizures

15. In general, the mechanisms of action of phenytoin-like agents are:

   A. desensitizing sodium channels in the CNS
   B. delaying the entry of potassium into neurons

   C. delaying the entry of calcium into neurons
   D. unknown

Matching—Terms and Definitions

Match the following vocabulary terms and their descriptions.

1. _____ Grand mal seizure

2. _____ Partial seizure

3. _____ Status epilepticus

4. _____ Tonic-clonic seizure

5. _____ Generalized seizure

A. Seizure originating and involving both cerebral hemispheres

B. An alternate contraction and relaxation of muscles, with a loss of consciousness, and abnormal behavior

C. Seizure originating in one area of the brain that may spread to other areas

D. Generalized seizure characterized by full-body tonic and clonic motor convulsions

E. An emergency situation characterized by continual seizure activity with no interruptions

Matching—Drug Names

Match the generic and trade names.

Generic Name

1. _____ primidone

2. _____ methsuximide

3. _____ carbamazepine

4. _____ valproic acid

5. _____ fosphenytoin

Trade Name

A. Cerebyx®

B. Tegretol®

C. Depakene®

D. Mysoline®

E. Celontin®

Fill in the Blank

Select terms from your reading to fill in the blanks.

1. Valproic acid is used cautiously in patients with a history of _____ disease or renal impairment.

2. Carbamazepine and valproic acid are classified as _____ drugs.

3. Hypoalbuminemia means _____ albumin in the blood plasma.

4. Fosphenytoin is converted to _____ in the body and is parenterally used for control of _____.

5. Barbiturates are classified as either Schedule _____ or _____ medications.

6. Generalized seizures have _____ foci that may cause loss of consciousness.

7. Seizure disorders are classified by their location in the _____ and their clinical features.

8. Seizure is a term for all _____ events.

9. More than 2,500 barbiturates have been synthesized, but only about _____ have been approved for clinical use in the United States.

10. Partial seizures have a _____ or _____ origin, often in the cerebral cortex.

11. 75% to 90% of seizure patients have their first seizure before age _____.

12. Antiseizure drugs _____ or stop a convulsive seizure.

13. Epilepsy is the _____ term for _____ seizures.

14. The international classification of seizures include partial seizures and _____ seizures.

15. Convulsion relates to _____ motor movements.

True or False

Select the letter "T" or "F" for the following questions.

____ 1. Infantile spasms are classified as partial or focal seizures.

____ 2. The terms *epilepsy, convulsions*, and *seizures* are commonly used interchangeably.

____ 3. Phenobarbital is used in seizure disorders.

____ 4. The trade name of diazepam is Klonopin®.

____ 5. Phenytoin may also cause dysrhythmias.

____ 6. Gingival hyperplasia is an adverse effect of phenobarbital sodium (Luminal®).

____ 7. The mechanism of action of phenytoin-like agents resembles the mechanism of action of phenytoin.

____ 8. Myoclonic means contraction and relaxation of the muscles.

____ 9. Serious injury or death can occur in patients with implanted neurologic stimulators who undergo magnetic resonance imaging (MRI) procedures.

____ 10. Clonazepam can also cause abnormal reduction of all circulating blood cells and vaginal bleeding.

ANSWER KEY

Multiple Choice

1. C	2. B	3. D	4. A	5. D
6. D	7. A	8. A	9. C	10. D
11. A	12. B	13. B	14. C	15. D

Matching—Terms and Definitions

1. D	2. C	3. E	4. B	5. A

Matching—Drug Names

1. D	2. E	3. B	4. C	5. A

Fill in the Blank

1. kidney	2. phenytoin-like	3. low
4. phenytoin; status epilepticus	5. II; III	6. multiple
7. brain	8. epileptic	9. 50
10. single; focal	11. 20	12. prevent
13. old; recurrent	14. generalized	15. abnormal

True or False

1. F	2. T	3. T	4. F	5. T
6. F	7. T	8. T	9. T	10. F

CHAPTER 9

Anesthetic Drugs

Multiple Choice

Select the correct answer from choices A–D.

1. Which of the following is the reason that chloroform is rarely used today?

   A. because of its expensiveness
   B. because of its toxicity
   C. because of its carcinogenic properties
   D. because of its ineffectiveness

2. All of the following medications are commonly used as preoperative drugs, except:

   A. opioid analgesics
   B. antianxiety agents
   C. anticholinergics
   D. antihistamine agents

3. The trade name of isoflurane is:

   A. Forane®
   B. Fluothane®
   C. Penthrane®
   D. Ultane®

4. Nitrous oxide provides analgesia equivalent to 10 mg of morphine, but may cause occasional episodes of:

   A. diarrhea and shortness of breath
   B. heartburn and headache
   C. nausea and vomiting
   D. hypertension and hot flashes

5. Which of the following drugs are used as intravenous anesthetics?

   A. barbiturates
   B. opioids
   C. benzodiazepines
   D. all of the above

6. The generic name of Ativan® is:

   A. lorazepam
   B. diazepam
   C. midazolam
   D. etomidate

7. Local anesthetics are mainly used in which of the following conditions?

   A. excision of superficial growths
   B. removal of cataracts
   C. removal of the gallbladder
   D. A and B

8. All of the following local anesthetics are classified as esters, except:

   A. cocaine
   B. dibucaine
   C. procaine
   D. benzocaine

9. Xylocaine® is the trade name of:

   A. procaine
   B. chloroprocaine

   C. lidocaine
   D. mepivacaine

10. All of the following ester-type local anesthetics have a rapid onset and short duration of activity, except:

   A. tetracaine
   B. procaine

   C. benzocaine
   D. cocaine

11. All of the following are the major routes for applying local anesthetics, except:

   A. spinal
   B. epidural

   C. subdural
   D. infiltration

12. *Hyperkalemia* means an increased number of which of the following ions in the blood?

   A. calcium
   B. potassium

   C. sodium
   D. magnesium

13. Which of the following is a serious adverse effect of inhalation anesthetics that must be treated immediately?

   A. malignant tumor
   B. malignant hypertension

   C. malignant hyperthermia
   D. A and B

14. The provision of a pain-free state for the entire body is referred to as:

   A. general anesthesia
   B. epidural anesthesia

   C. infiltration anesthesia
   D. all of the above

15. For several centuries, which of the following agents were the mainstays of anesthetics in the control of pain?

   A. barbiturates
   B. chloroform and nitrous oxide

   C. alcohol and opiates
   D. cocaine and benzodiazepines

16. Each of the following is a stage of general anesthesia, except:

   A. delirium
   B. medullary paralysis

   C. cessation of respiration
   D. amnesia and analgesia

17. Injectable anesthetics are used for which of the following reasons?

   A. to reduce the dose of an inhaled drug
   B. to reduce recovery time

   C. to provide more analgesia
   D. A and C

18. Amidate® is the trade name of:

   A. propofol
   B. etomidate

   C. diazepam
   D. alfentanil

19. Which of the following is an example of a topical anesthetic agent?

   A. ketamine hydrochloride
   B. enflurane

   C. lidocaine
   D. lorazepam

20. Which of the following statements is true?

   A. Preanesthetic and adjunct drugs are given before surgery.
   B. Preanesthetic and adjunct drugs are given during surgery.

   C. Preanesthetic and adjunct drugs are given after surgery.
   D. All of these statements are true.

Matching—Drugs and Uses

Match the numbered drug to its lettered description.

Drug	Use
1. _____ desflurane	A. used alone in dentistry and obstetrics
2. _____ methoxyflurane	B. used for epidural; has a short duration of action
3. _____ benzocaine	C. local anesthetic and antiarrhythmic drug
4. _____ chloroprocaine	D. used during labor; does not suppress uterine contractions
5. _____ lidocaine	E. used as a topical
6. _____ nitrous oxide	F. for induction and maintenance of general anesthesia

Matching—Drug Names

Match the generic and trade names.

Generic Name	Trade Name
1. _____ bupivacaine	A. Naropin®
2. _____ procaine	B. Carbocaine®
3. _____ mepivacaine	C. Xylocaine®
4. _____ prilocaine	D. Citanest®
5. _____ lidocaine	E. Novocain®
6. _____ ropivacaine	F. Marcaine®

Fill in the Blank

Select terms from your reading to fill in the blanks.

1. The two major groups of local anesthetics are _____ and _____.

2. *Lipophilic* means a substance is able to dissolve much more easily in _____ than in _____.

3. Injection of an anesthetic into the space immediately outside of the dura mater is referred to as _____ anesthesia.

4. Anesthesia is basically characterized by four reversible actions: unconsciousness, _____, immobility, and _____.

5. Volatile liquids evaporate upon exposure to the _____.

6. Stage 1 general anesthesia is characterized by: _____, _____, perceptual distortions, and amnesia.

7. The most potent of volatile agents is _____.

8. Stage IV is characterized by medullary paralysis, which begins with _____ failure, and can lead to circulatory collapse.

9. Laughing gas is also known as _____.

10. Inhaled general anesthetics are contraindicated in patients who have received monoamine oxidase inhibitors within the previous _____ days.

11. Inhaled general anesthetics should be used cautiously during pregnancy and in children younger than _____.

12. Intravenous anesthetics are often administered with _____ general anesthetics.

13. The amides have several _____ over the esters.

14. Ester-type local anesthetics have been in use _____ than amides.

15. Local anesthetics are used for _____.

16. The term "nystagmus" means rhythmical oscillation of the _____.

17. _____ anesthesia is probably the most common route used to administer local anesthetics.

18. _____ is a popular choice for infiltration anesthesia, but bupivacaine is used for longer procedures.

19. Malignant hyperthermia may cause the death of the patient due to _____ damage.

20. Malignant hyperthermia is characterized by severe overproduction of body _____ with rigidity of _____.

True or False

Select the letter "T" or "F" for the following questions.

____ 1. Epidural anesthesia involves injection of the local anesthetic in the lumbar or caudal areas.

____ 2. Dantrolene has a very short shelf life and must be restocked regularly.

____ 3. Local anesthetics are contraindicated in patients with severe hemorrhage, hypotension, and shock.

____ 4. Burning energy and nutrients at a higher rate than normal is called hypometabolism.

____ 5. Surgical anesthesia lasts until spontaneous respiration ceases.

____ 6. Stage II of general anesthesia is further divided into four planes.

____ 7. Stage III is characterized by progressive muscular contraction.

____ 8. Inhaled general anesthetics are all very lipophilic.

____ 9. Nitrous oxide at higher doses causes calmness and sedation.

____ 10. Most of the local anesthetics in common use today belong to the ester type.

ANSWER KEY

Multiple Choice

1. B	2. D	3. A	4. C	5. D
6. A	7. D	8. B	9. C	10. A
11. C	12. B	13. C	14. A	15. C
16. C	17. D	18. B	19. C	20. D

Matching—Drugs and Indications

1. F	2. D	3. E	4. B	5. C
6. A				

Matching—Drug Names

1. F	2. E	3. B	4. D	5. C
6. A				

Fill in the Blank

1. esters; amides	2. lipids; water	3. epidural	4. analgesia; amnesia
5. air	6. analgesia; euphoria	7. halothane	8. respiratory
9. nitrous oxide	10. fourteen	11. twelve	12. inhaled
13. advantages	14. longer	15. minor surgery	16. eyeballs
17. Local infiltration	18. Lidocaine	19. brain	20. heat; skeletal muscles

True or False

1. T	2. T	3. T	4. F	5. T
6. F	7. F	8. T	9. F	10. F

CHAPTER 10

Drug Therapy for the Musculoskeletal System

Multiple Choice

Select the correct answer from choices A–D.

1. Arthritis characterized by the erosion of articular cartilage that mainly affects weight-bearing joints in older adults is called:

   A. rheumatoid arthritis
   B. osteoporosis
   C. osteomalacia
   D. osteoarthritis

2. A hereditary metabolic form of acute arthritis is referred to as:

   A. bursitis
   B. gout
   C. Paget's disease
   D. scoliosis

3. An example of a synarthrosis joint is found in which of the following?

   A. the skull
   B. the pubic symphysis
   C. the shoulder
   D. the elbow

4. All of the following are among joints most commonly affected by rheumatoid arthritis, except:

   A. the vertebral column (lumbar region)
   B. the hands
   C. the knees
   D. the fingers

5. Which of the following is the mechanism of action of neuromuscular blocking agents?

   A. prevent sensory nerve impulses
   B. prevent motor nerve impulses
   C. inhibit autonomic nerve impulses
   D. all of the above

6. The principal use of neuromuscular blocking drugs is to:

   A. control respiration
   B. help orthopedic manipulation
   C. provide adequate skeletal muscular relaxation during surgery
   D. accomplish all of the above

7. Which of the following is the exact mechanism of centrally acting skeletal muscle relaxants?

   A. unknown
   B. prevent somatic motor nerve impulses
   C. suppress or prevent inflammation of skeletal muscle
   D. inhibit the release of acetylcholine

8. Common adverse effects of gold compounds include which of the following?

   A. blindness
   B. advanced rheumatoid arthritis

   C. lesions of the mucous membranes, and dermatitis
   D. increased occurrence of seizures in patients with epilepsy

9. All of the following are centrally acting skeletal muscle relaxants, except:

   A. baclofen
   B. chlorphenesin

   C. allopurinol
   D. methocarbamol

10. Robaxin® is the trade name of:

    A. baclofen
    B. chlorphenesin

    C. allopurinol
    D. methocarbamol

11. Dantrolene is an example of which of the following classes of drugs?

    A. centrally acting skeletal muscle relaxants
    B. direct acting skeletal muscle relaxants

    C. loop diuretics
    D. antihypertensives

12. A stretching or a partial tear in a muscle or a muscle-tendon unit is called a:

    A. strain
    B. sprain

    C. stress
    D. none of the above

13. All of the following are types of joints, except:

    A. diarthrosis
    B. synarthrosis

    C. amphiarthrosis
    D. aphthosis

14. A specialized junction at which a nerve cell communicates with a target cell is referred to as a:

    A. neuron
    B. synapse

    C. synaptic cleft
    D. neuromuscular junction

15. Which of the following is a waste product of purine metabolism?

    A. calcium sulfate
    B. ketone bodies

    C. uric acid
    D. carbonic acid

16. All of the following are adverse effects of long-term administration of corticosteroids, except:

    A. osteoarthritis
    B. osteoporosis

    C. hypertension
    D. hyperglycemia

17. Colchicine is often combined with which of the following agents to improve prophylactic therapy of chronic gouty arthritis?

    A. methotrexate
    B. probenecid

    C. penicillamine
    D. penicillin

18. Which of the following is not an analgesic?

    A. diazepam
    B. gold sodium thiomalate

    C. auranofin
    D. allopurinol

19. Which of the following agents is most effective to relieve pain and inflammation for acute gout attack when initiated 12 to 36 hours after symptoms begin?

    A. colchicine
    B. allopurinol

    C. penicillamine
    D. prednisone

20. The peak incidence of rheumatoid arthritis among women is between the ages of:

    A. 15-25 years
    B. 30-50 years

    C. 40-60 years
    D. 70-90 years

Matching—Terms and Descriptions

Match the lettered term to its numbered description.

_____ 1. Injury to supporting ligaments of a joint   A. Rheumatoid arthritis

_____ 2. A disease caused by deposits of uric acid in the big toe   B. Osteoarthritis

_____ 3. Inflammation of articular cartilage that mainly affects weight-bearing   C. Gout
joints in older adults

_____ 4. Injury resulting from overstretching of a muscle; it results in tearing   D. Strain
of the muscle or muscle and tendon

_____ 5. A chronic and progressive condition leading to deformity and   E. Sprain
disability

Matching—Drug Names

Match the generic and trade names.

Generic Name		Trade Name
_____ 1.	pancuronium	A. Lioresal®
_____ 2.	botulinum toxin type B	B. Dantrium®
_____ 3.	mivacurium	C. Soma®
_____ 4.	penicillamine	D. Ridaura®
_____ 5.	cyclobenzaprine	E. Azulfidine®
_____ 6.	auranofin	F. Depen®
_____ 7.	sulfasalazine	G. Myoblock®
_____ 8.	dantrolene	H. Flexeril®
_____ 9.	carisoprodol	I. Mivacron®
_____ 10.	baclofen	J. Pavulon®

Fill in the Blank

Select terms from your reading to fill in the blanks.

1. Most skeletal injuries are accompanied by _____ injuries.

2. The cause of rheumatoid arthritis is _____.

3. Gout often affects a _____ joint.

4. Examples of neuromuscular blocking agents include succinylcholine, atracurium, and _____.

5. Baclofen (a centrally acting muscle relaxant) is often the drug of first choice because of
its _____.

6. Dantrolene should be used cautiously in patients younger than _____ (especially women).

7. The mechanism of action of penicillamine is _____.

8. Inflammation of the joints is called _____.

9. In acute gout, immobilization of the affected joint is _____.

10. Colchicine is a gout suppressant with antimitotic and indirect _____ properties.

11. Allopurinol is contraindicated in _____, except those with hyperuricemia secondary
to _____.

12. Skeletal muscle allows _____ movement.

13. The muscular system consists of three types of muscle: skeletal, _____, and _____.

14. The skeletal system consists of _____ bones.

15. Neuromuscular blocking agents are not effective for rigidity and spasticity of muscles caused by _____ disease or trauma.

True or False

____ 1. A cut or break in the skin is called a contusion.

____ 2. The term "articular" is related to the skeletal muscle of the body.

____ 3. Spasticity is a type of increase in muscle tone at rest.

____ 4. An example of a diarthrosis is found in the knee or elbow.

____ 5. Cardiac muscle can be controlled by the wishes of the individual.

____ 6. The most common causes of childhood injuries are falls and sports injuries.

____ 7. Relaxation of skeletal muscle occurs when acetylcholine is broken down by calcium and vitamin D.

____ 8. Cycoflex® is the trade name of cyclobenzaprine.

____ 9. Quinine sulfate is also used to treat malignant hyperthermia.

____ 10. Corticosteroids do not alter the course of rheumatoid arthritis.

ANSWER KEY

Multiple Choice

1. D	2. B	3. A	4. A	5. B
6. D	7. A	8. C	9. C	10. D
11. B	12. A	13. D	14. B	15. C
16. A	17. B	18. D	19. A	20. C

Matching—Terms and Descriptions

1. E	2. C	3. B	4. D	5. A

Matching—Drug Names

1. J	2. G	3. I	4. F	5. H
6. D	7. E	8. B	9. C	10. A

Fill in the Blank

1. soft tissue	2. unknown	3. single
4. doxacurium	5. wide safety margin	6. 35 years
7. unknown	8. arthritis	9. essential
10. anti-inflammatory	11. children; cancer	12. voluntary
13. smooth; cardiac	14. 206	15. neurological

True or False

1. F	2. F	3. T	4. T	5. F
6. T	7. F	8. T	9. F	10. T

CHAPTER 11

Drug Therapy for Cardiovascular Disorders

Multiple Choice

Select the correct answer from choices A–D.

1. Which of the following are the smallest type of blood vessels?

   A. veins
   B. arteries
   C. arterioles
   D. capillaries

2. Degenerative changes in small arteries, which commonly occur in older individuals and diabetics, are referred to as:

   A. silent angina
   B. arteriosclerosis
   C. atherosclerosis
   D. atheromas

3. Which of the following is a calcium channel blocker?

   A. metoprolol (Lopressor®)
   B. timolol (Betimol®)
   C. bepridil (Vascor®)
   D. propranolol (Inderal®)

4. Which of the following factors may increase the shelf life of nitroglycerin?

   A. storing it in a refrigerator in a tightly closed container
   B. storing it in a dark, tightly closed container
   C. keeping it out of reach of children
   D. both A and C

5. Abrupt discontinuation of long-acting nitroglycerin preparations may cause:

   A. blindness
   B. stroke
   C. angina
   D. hypertension

6. Beta-blockers decrease the effects of the sympathetic nervous system by blocking the release of which of the following neurotransmitters?

   A. dopamine
   B. epinephrine
   C. acetylcholine
   D. none of the above

7. Calcium channel blockers are used to treat which of the following types of angina that is not controlled by nitrates?

   A. exertional angina
   B. silent angina
   C. vasospastic angina
   D. all of the above

8. Myocardial infarction is produced by which of the following?

   A. An obstruction of the small intestine
   B. An obstruction of the small arteries in the brain
   C. An obstruction of the small vein
   D. An obstruction of the coronary artery

9. When the heart beats between 150 and 250 times per minute, the condition is referred to as:

   A. bradycardia
   B. tachycardia
   C. atrial fibrillation
   D. ventricular fibrillation

10. Which of the following is the class of sodium channel blockers?

    A. Class I
    B. Class II
    C. Class III
    D. Class IV

11. Which of the following is an example of Class IV antiarrhythmic drugs?

    A. propranolol (Inderal®)
    B. amiodarone (Cordarone®)
    C. verapamil (Calan®)
    D. lidocaine (Xylocaine®)

12. Which of the following is the trade name of nadolol?

    A. Brevibloc®
    B. Corgard®
    C. Sectral®
    D. Tenormin®

13. Which of the following are one of the oldest types of drugs used in the treatment of heart diseases?

    A. calcium channel blockers
    B. sodium channel blockers
    C. potassium channel blockers
    D. cardiac glycosides

14. Which of the following is the principal medication for the treatment of congestive heart failure?

    A. digitalis
    B. a calcium channel blocker
    C. a β-blocker
    D. all of the above

15. Nocturnal angina can be treated by which of the following medications?

    A. calcium channel blockers
    B. digitalis
    C. nitrates
    D. A and C

16. Decubitus angina is characterized by periodic attacks of cardiac pain that occur when a person is:

    A. running
    B. lying down
    C. getting angry
    D. eating

17. Which of the following statements is not true regarding unstable angina?

    A. It typically has a sudden onset and sudden worsening
    B. It has a more severe short-term prognosis than stable chronic angina
    C. It occurs in the absence of angina pain
    D. It occurs during periods of rest

18. All of the following are groups of medications that may meet the treatment goals for angina pectoris, except:

    A. calcium channel blockers
    B. potassium channel blockers
    C. β-adrenergic blockers
    D. Nitrates

19. In bradycardia, the heart beats:

    A. less than 60 times per minute
    B. 100 to 200 times per minute
    C. 200 to 350 times per minute
    D. more than 350 times per minute

20. Which of the following sub-classifications of antiarrhythmic agents are listed as Class II?

    A. calcium channel blockers
    B. fast channel blockers
    C. β-adrenergic blockers
    D. none of the above

Matching—Terms and Descriptions

Match the lettered term to its numbered description.

Description	Antiarrhythmic Agent
_____ 1. Selectively block slow calcium channels	A. Class I
_____ 2. Decrease fast sodium influx to cardiac cells	B. Class II
_____ 3. Inhibit adrenergic stimulation of the heart, and depress myocardial excitability and contractility	C. Class III
_____ 4. Interfere with potassium outflow during repolarization	D. Class IV

Matching—Drug Names

Match the generic and trade names.

Generic Name	Trade Name
_____ 1. verapamil	A. Tambocor®
_____ 2. esmolol	B. Norpace®
_____ 3. flecainide	C. Ethmozine®
_____ 4. propafenone	D. Rythmol®
_____ 5. disopyramide	E. Brevibloc®
_____ 6. moricizine	F. Calan®

Fill in the Blank

Select terms from your reading to fill in the blanks.

1. The heart is a hollow muscular organ consisting of the endocardium, pericardium, and _____.

2. Atherosclerotic lesions that produce a narrowing of the coronary arteries are the major cause of _____.

3. There are several types of angina: stable (classic), unstable, decubitus (nocturnal), and _____ angina.

4. The largest of the blood vessels are the _____.

5. Nitrates were the first agents used to _____.

6. After a container of nitroglycerin is opened, the drug is effective for approximately _____ months.

7. Myocardial infarction is produced by an obstruction of the _____ arteries.

8. Digitalis drugs are the principal medications for the treatment of congestive heart failure and certain _____.

9. A procedure wherein a vein graft is surgically implanted to bypass part of an occlusion in a coronary artery is called a coronary arterial _____.

10. The veins carry deoxygenated blood away from the _____ to the heart.

11. Digoxin is prescribed most frequently because it can be administered orally and _____.

12. The cardiovascular system consists of the heart, blood vessels, _____, and _____.

13. Myocardial infarction is an area of _____ cardiac muscle tissue.

14. During acute myocardial infarction, women are less likely to experience _____ than men.

15. There are two circuits for blood flow: the pulmonary circuit and the _____ circuit.

16. Quinidine is used to treat supraventricular _____.

17. The myocardium conducts its own electrical impulses, which serve to regulate the _____.

18. The most dangerous adverse effect of digoxin is its ability to cause dysrhythmias, particularly in patients who have _____.

19. Arrhythmias reduce the efficiency of the heart's _____ cycle.

20. Cardiac glycosides act by increasing the _____ and velocity of myocardial systolic contraction.

True or False

Select the letter "T" or "F" for the following questions.

____ 1. Plaques consisting of lipids, cells, and cell debris, often with attached thrombi, that form inside the walls of large arteries are referred to as *thrombi*.

____ 2. Silent angina is a condition that occurs in the absence of chest pain.

____ 3. The main functions of the lymphatic system include: the returning of excess fluid from tissues to the circulatory system, and the manufacture of lymphocytes.

____ 4. Nitrates are used in the treatment of angina as coronary vasoconstrictors.

____ 5. Beta-blockers are the newest type of drugs that block the entry of calcium into smooth muscle cells.

____ 6. Chest pain relief in myocardial infarction is best achieved with oxygen, nitroglycerin, and morphine sulfate.

____ 7. Antithrombotic agents should be considered for all patients with an acute myocardial infarction.

____ 8. There are five subgroups of fast channel blockers.

____ 9. Examples of Class IA antiarrhythmic drugs are atropine, magnesium, and digoxin.

____ 10. Examples of Class IV agents (calcium channel blockers) include verapamil (Calan®) and diltiazem (Cardizem®).

ANSWER KEY

Multiple Choice

1. D	2. B	3. C	4. B	5. C
6. B	7. A	8. D	9. B	10. A
11. C	12. B	13. D	14. A	15. D
16. B	17. C	18. B	19. A	20. C

Matching—Terms and Descriptions

1. D	2. A	3. B	4. C

Matching—Drug Names

1. F	2. E	3. A	4. D	5. B	6. C

Fill in the Blank

1. myocardium	2. angina	3. silent
4. arteries	5. relieve angina	6. six
7. coronary	8. arrhythmias	9. bypass graft
10. capillaries	11. parenterally	12. blood; lymph
13. dead	14. chest pain	15. systemic
16. arrhythmias	17. heartbeat	18. hypokalemia
19. pumping	20. force	

True or False

1. F	2. T	3. T	4. F	5. F
6. T	7. T	8. F	9. F	10. T

CHAPTER 12

Antihypertensive Agents and Hyperlipidemia

Multiple Choice

Select the correct answer from choices A–D.

1. Essential hypertension develops when the blood pressure is consistently above which of the following?

    A. 110/80
    B. 120/85

    C. 130/90
    D. 140/90

2. Which of the following types of drugs are not antihypertensive medications?

    A. angiotensin-converting enzyme inhibitors
    B. angiotensin I receptor antagonists

    C. adrenergic blockers
    D. peripheral vasodilators

3. Which of the following drugs are becoming the drugs of choice in the first-line treatment of essential hypertension?

    A. angiotensin-converting enzyme inhibitors
    B. centrally and peripherally acting blockers

    C. diuretics
    D. peripheral vasodilators

4. Which of the following is not the mechanism of action of angiotensin II receptor antagonist drugs?

    A. blocking the binding of angiotensin I to the angiotensin II receptors
    B. blocking the binding of angiotensin II to the angiotensin I receptors

    C. blocking the binding of angiotensin II to the angiotensin II receptors
    D. none of the above

5. Which of the following diuretics are the most commonly used to treat essential hypertension?

    A. loop diuretics
    B. thiazide diuretics

    C. potassium-sparing diuretics
    D. none of the above

6. Which of the following conditions or disorders may produce a life-threatening elevation of triglycerides?

    A. pneumonia
    B. meningitis

    C. pancreatitis
    D. nephritis

7. Which of the following is known as "good cholesterol"?

    A. LDL
    B. VLDL

    C. HDL
    D. triglyceride

8. Which of the following is not an HMG-CoA reductase inhibitor (statin)?

    A. Zocor®
    B. Atromid-S®

    C. Lipitor®
    D. Mevacor®

9. The statin drugs are used as adjuncts to diet when which of the following is elevated?

   A. total cholesterol
   B. LDL cholesterol

   C. serum triglycerides
   D. all of the above

10. The sympatholytic drugs include all of the following groups of medications, except:

   A. centrally acting alpha-antagonists
   B. postganglionic adrenergic blockers

   C. beta-adrenergic agonist agents
   D. alpha-adrenergic blocking agents

11. Which of the following agents are used for the initial treatment of hypertension?

   A. beta-blockers
   B. diuretics

   C. antibiotics
   D. HMG-CoA reductase inhibitors

12. Bile acid sequestrants increase the action of which of the following?

   A. loss of normal liver cells
   B. loss of bile acids

   C. serum cholesterol levels
   D. serum triglycerides

13. All of the following agents are peripherally acting blockers, except:

   A. guanethidine (Ismelin®)
   B. prazosin (Minipress®)

   C. methyldopa (Aldomet®)
   D. terazosin (Hytrin®)

14. The causes of secondary hypertension include all of the following, except:

   A. hyperaldosteronism
   B. hypocholesterolemia

   C. pheochromocytoma
   D. nephrosclerosis

15. The areas most commonly damaged from severe hypertension include all of the following, except:

   A. bone marrow
   B. kidneys

   C. retinas
   D. brain

16. Beta-blockers reduce peripheral resistance and inhibit cardiac function. They also block secretion of which of the following substances:

   A. insulin
   B. erythropoietin

   C. aldosterone
   D. renin

17. Which of the following is a true statement regarding vasodilators?

   A. Vasodilators block the movement of potassium into the smooth muscle of arteries
   B. Vasodilators are prescribed as second-line agents to initial therapy for hypertension

   C. Vasodilators are reducers of hypotension
   D. All of the above

18. Patients taking guanethidine should avoid over-the-counter preparations that contain adrenergic substances, because the combination may potentiate an acute hypertensive effect. Which of the following contains adrenergic substances?

   A. cold medicines
   B. vitamin B_{12} and niacin

   C. aspirin or acetaminophen
   D. milk of magnesia

19. Minipress® is the trade name of:

   A. furosemide
   B. spironolactone

   C. prazosin
   D. chlorothiazide

20. Which of the following is the mechanism of action for fibric acid derivatives?

   A. Stimulation of the liver to increase breakdown of VLDL to HDL and increase liver synthesis of VLDL to HDL
   B. Stimulation of the liver to increase breakdown of HDL to LDL and increase liver synthesis of HDL to LDL

   C. Stimulation of the liver to increase breakdown of VLDL to LDL and decrease liver synthesis of VLDL by inhibiting cholesterol formation
   D. None of the above

Matching—Terms and Descriptions

Match the lettered term to its numbered description.

Description

_____ 1. The amount of blood pumped with each heartbeat

_____ 2. Hardening of blood vessels

_____ 3. Known as idiopathic hypertension

_____ 4. Results from renal or endocrine disorders

_____ 5. The amount of blood the heart pumps to the body in one minute

_____ 6. Severe and rapidly progressive form of hypertension

Term

A. Primary hypertension

B. Cardiac output

C. Malignant hypertension

D. Sclerotic

E. Secondary hypertension

F. Stroke volume

Matching—Drug Names

Match the generic and trade names.

Generic Name

_____ 1. irbesartan

_____ 2. metoprolol

_____ 3. guanadrel

_____ 4. prazosin

_____ 5. spironolactone

_____ 6. diazoxide

_____ 7. minoxidil

_____ 8. clonidine

Trade Name

A. Catapres®

B. Hyperstat®

C. Rogaine®

D. Aldactone®

E. Minipress®

F. Lopressor®

G. Hylorel®

H. Avapro®

Fill in the Blank

Select terms from your reading to fill in the blanks.

1. Hydralazine and minoxidil may be used in the treatment of moderate essential or early _____ hypertension.

2. Vasodilators block the movement of calcium into the _____ muscle of the blood vessels to cause _____ of the muscle.

3. Beta-blockers should be used with caution in patients with hepatic or _____ impairment.

4. Diuretics increase _____ excretion and lower blood volume.

5. Diamox® is used to lower _____ pressure.

6. Antihyperlipidemic drugs are used only if _____ modification and _____ programs fail to lower LDL to normal levels.

7. Niacin is used cautiously in individuals with history of gallbladder disease, liver impairment, and _____.

8. Loop diuretics inhibit sodium and chloride _____.

9. Cholestyramine (Questran®) and colestipol (Colestid®) are examples of _____ sequestrants.

10. Thiazide agents increase the excretion of water, _____, chloride, and _____.

11. Angiotensin-converting enzyme (ACE) inhibitors slow the formation of _____, which reduces vascular resistance.

12. The primary indication of clofibrate is for _____ that does not respond to diet.

13. Alpha and beta blockers are used for _____ patients who have not responded to initial antihypertensive therapy.

14. Normal systolic blood pressure in adults is less than _____ mg Hg.

15. A blood chemical whose molecules are comprised of a lipid portion and a protein portion is known as a _____.

16. The most important site of angiotensin-converting enzyme (ACE) is in the _____, but ACE also is found in the kidneys.

17. Niacin (vitamin B_3) can exert _____ and _____ lowering effects at high dosages.

18. Peripherally acting adrenergic inhibitors are powerful _____ agents.

19. Beta blockers _____ peripheral resistance and inhibit cardiac function.

20. Mannitol and urea are most commonly used to reduce _____ or intraocular pressure.

True or False

Select the letter "T" or "F" for the following questions.

____ 1. Blood pressure is determined by cardiac output and stroke volume.

____ 2. When hypertension is not properly treated, the risk of peptic ulcer and pneumonia increases.

____ 3. Lower angiotensin II levels increase plasma renin activity and reduce aldosterone secretion.

____ 4. Centrally acting blockers include clonidine (Catapres®) and methyldopa (Aldomet®).

____ 5. Excess fat in the blood is called "hyperglycemia."

____ 6. Antihyperlipidemics are used to decrease the risk of blood clotting.

____ 7. The trade name of lovastatin is Lipitor®.

____ 8. The type of diuretic used is determined by the condition being treated.

____ 9. Propranolol was the first beta-blocking agent shown to block both $beta_1$ and $beta_2$ receptors.

____ 10. The angiotensin II class of drugs was the first class used for the treatment of hypertension.

ANSWER KEY

Multiple Choice

1. D	2. B	3. A	4. B	5. B
6. C	7. C	8. B	9. D	10. C
11. A	12. B	13. C	14. B	15. A
16. D	17. B	18. A	19. C	20. C

Matching—Terms and Descriptions

1. F	2. D	3. A	4. E	5. B	6. C

Matching—Drug Names

1. H	2. F	3. G	4. E	5. D
6. B	7. C	8. A		

Fill in the Blank

1. malignant	2. smooth; relaxation	3. renal
4. sodium	5. intraocular	6. diet; exercise
7. peptic ulcer	8. reabsorption	9. bile acid
10. sodium; potassium	11. angiotensin II	12. hyperlipidemia
13. hypertensive	14. 120	15. lipoprotein
16. lungs	17. cholesterol; triglyceride	18. antihypertensive
19. reduce	20. intracranial	

True or False

1. T	2. F	3. T	4. T	5. F
6. F	7. F	8. T	9. T	10. F

CHAPTER 13

Anticoagulant Drugs

Multiple Choice

Select the correct answer from choices A–D.

1. Which of the following cells contains histamine?

   A. eosinophils
   B. erythrocytes

   C. mast cells
   D. neutrophils

2. A process that stops bleeding in a blood vessel is called:

   A. hematoma
   B. hemostasis

   C. hemopoiesis
   D. hemolysis

3. Thrombin is:

   A. an enzyme
   B. an acid

   C. a hormone
   D. a mineral

4. The immediate response of a blood vessel to injury is:

   A. the release of thromboplastin
   B. the changing of fibrinogen into fibrin

   C. the release of heparin at the site of injury
   D. vasoconstriction

5. The indications of heparin include which of the following conditions?

   A. pneumothorax
   B. pulmonary embolism

   C. pneumoconiosis
   D. pneumonia

6. All of the following agents are classified as low molecular weight (fractionated) heparins, except:

   A. dalteparin (Fragmin®)
   B. tinzaparin (Innohep®)

   C. enoxaparin (Lovenox®)
   D. anisindione (Miradon®)

7. Which of the following drugs is an anticoagulant?

   A. lepirudin (Refludan®)
   B. eptifibatide (Integrilin®)

   C. ticlopidine (Ticlid®)
   D. anistreplase (Eminase®)

8. Which of the following is the most common adverse effect of thrombolytic drugs?

   A. hemorrhoid
   B. hepatitis

   C. bleeding
   D. bone marrow depression

9. Antiplatelet drugs are used cautiously in patients with:

   A. severe liver and renal impairment
   B. surgery

   C. stroke
   D. A and B

10. Which of the following agents prevents platelet aggregation?

    A. tinzaparin (Innohep®)   C. enoxaparin (Lovenox®)
    B. ticlopidine (Ticlid®)   D. heparin sodium (Hep-Lock®)

11. Thrombophlebitis refers to the development of a thrombus in which of the following blood vessels?

    A. veins   C. arterioles
    B. arteries   D. B and C

12. Which of the following is the generic name for Coumadin®?

    A. heparin sodium   C. warfarin
    B. lepirudin   D. enoxaparin

13. Which of the following is the major complication of heparin administration?

    A. pruritus   C. spontaneous bleeding
    B. hypertension   D. chest pain

14. Which of the following is the mainstay of long-term anticoagulant therapy?

    A. heparin sodium   C. enoxaparin
    B. warfarin   D. lepirudin

15. The most commonly used antiplatelet drug is:

    A. eptifibatide   C. abciximab
    B. dipyridamole   D. aspirin

16. Which of the following is the generic name for Abbokinase®?

    A. urokinase   C. anistreplase
    B. streptokinase   D. reteplase recombinant

17. Warfarin is structurally similar to which of the following?

    A. heparin sodium   C. vitamin C
    B. aspirin   D. vitamin K

18. Which of the following the trade name of abciximab?

    A. Persantine®   C. Aggrastat®
    B. ReoPro®   D. Plavix®

19. Which of the following is a glycoprotein formed and stored in the parenchymal cells of the liver and present in the blood?

    A. thrombosis   C. thrombus
    B. thrombin   D. prothrombin

20. Which of the following anticoagulant drugs is given orally?

    A. warfarin sodium   C. enoxaparin
    B. heparin sodium   D. lepirudin

Matching—Drug Names

Match the generic and trade names.

Generic Name   Trade Name

_____ 1. pentoxifylline   A. Coumadin®

_____ 2. clopidogrel   B. ASA®

_____ 3. argatroban   C. Integrilin®

_____ 4. eptifibatide   D. Angiomax®

_____ 5. tinzaparin   E. Eminase®

_____ 6. alteplase recombinant   F. Activase®

_____ 7. anistreplase   G. Plavix®

_____ 8. aspirin   H. Innohep®

_____ 9. bivalirudin   I. Acova®

_____ 10. warfarin   J. Trental®

Fill in the Blank

Select terms from your reading to fill in the blanks.

1. Blood coagulation is of the utmost importance in the protection of the body from undue blood _____.

2. Thromboplastin and calcium react with prothrombin to create _____.

3. Thrombin changes fibrinogen into _____.

4. Vitamin K _____ may cause a _____ in prothrombin and fibrinogen levels.

5. Hemophilia causes bleeding disorders resulting from a deficiency of one of the _____.

6. Anticoagulants are used to prevent _____ clots from forming.

7. In humans, heparin is usually found in _____ or mast cells.

8. Heparin may be administered _____ to patients at risk for thrombus formation.

9. Heparin can be inactivated by hydrochloric acid in the _____.

10. Low molecular weight heparins have become the drugs of choice for many _____ disorders.

11. Heparin can be discontinued after about _____, as the oral anticoagulants take this much time to exert their effect.

12. The low molecular weight heparins may produce _____ adverse effects.

13. Alopecia and sustained erection are the only adverse effects of any consequence of _____.

14. Antiplatelet agents are prescribed to suppress aggregation of _____.

15. The term "aggregation" means the _____ together of platelets to form a _____.

16. Substances causing blood clots are called _____.

17. Heparin and heparin substitutes are used _____ for deep vein, pulmonary, or atrial embolism.

18. Cholestyramine can _____ warfarin absorption, thus reducing its effects.

19. Clopidogrel is an _____ agent used in patients who have recently had myocardial infarction or stroke.

20. Plasmin is an enzyme that breaks down the _____ of a blood clot.

True or False

Select the letter "T" or "F" for the following questions.

____ 1. The body normally regulates fibrinolysis such that unwanted fibrin clots are removed.

____ 2. Antiplatelets should be avoided in patients with recent major surgery.

____ 3. Abciximab is an antiplatelet drug used with acetaminophen to prevent fever and constipation.

____ 4. The primary side effects associated with glycoprotein antagonists are clotting and thrombocytosis.

____ 5. Urokinase is capable of dissolving an arterial clot.

____ 6. Thrombolytic drugs are used to treat acute ischemic cerebrovascular accident.

____ 7. Warfarin is used as an adjunct in the treatment of coronary occlusion and cerebral transient ischemic attacks.

____ 8. Warfarin is used cautiously in psychosis.

____ 9. Heparin preparations are used with caution in patients with alcoholism or asthma.

____ 10. Vitamin K deficiency may cause an increase in prothrombin and fibrinogen levels.

ANSWER KEY

Multiple Choice

1. C	2. B	3. A	4. D	5. B
6. D	7. A	8. C	9. D	10. B
11. A	12. C	13. C	14. B	15. D
16. A	17. D	18. B	19. D	20. A

Matching—Drug Names

1. L	2. G	3. I	4. C	5. H
6. F	7. E	8. B	9. D	10. A

Fill in the Blank

1. loss	2. thrombin	3. fibrin	4. deficiency; decrease
5. clotting factors	6. new	7. basophils	8. intravenously
9. stomach	10. clotting	11. 48 hours	12. fewer
13. warfarin	14. platelets	15. clumping; clot	16. thrombogenic
17. prophylactically	18. decrease	19. antiplatelet	20. fibrin

True or False

1. T	2. T	3. F	4. F	5. T
6. T	7. T	8. T	9. T	10. F

CHAPTER 14

Drug Therapy for Allergies and Respiratory Disorders

Multiple Choice

Select the correct answer from choices A–D.

1. The term "antigen" means:

   A. a chemical substance naturally found in all body tissues
   B. an agent that promotes the removal of mucus secretions from the lungs
   C. a substance that is introduced into the body and causes white blood cells to react
   D. a substance that releases lymphocytes

2. The lower respiratory system consists of all of the following, except:

   A. trachea
   B. pharynx
   C. bronchioles
   D. alveoli

3. Which of the following chemical substances may be released from mast cells, platelets, and basophils?

   A. norepinephrine
   B. antibody
   C. renin
   D. histamine

4. Emphysema involves the destruction of the:

   A. trachea
   B. alveolar air space
   C. bronchi
   D. bronchioles

5. Which of the following is the generic name for Benadryl®?

   A. clemastine fumarate
   B. promethazine hydrochloride
   C. diphenhydramine hydrochloride
   D. triprolidine hydrochloride

6. Which of the following agents are used to treat minor symptoms of various allergic conditions and the common cold?

   A. H_1-receptor agonists
   B. H_1-receptor antagonists
   C. H_2-receptor antagonists
   D. H_2-receptor agonists

7. Which of the following is not an anti-inflammatory medication for the treatment of asthma?

   A. fluticasone (Flovent®)
   B. flunisolide (AeroBid®)
   C. salmeterol (Serevent®)
   D. triamcinolone (Azmacort®)

8. Xanthine derivatives are contraindicated in which of the following conditions or disorders?

   A. hyperthyroidism
   B. asthma
   C. emphysema
   D. bronchitis

9. Systematic glucocorticoids are used to treat:

   A. viral infections
   B. active tuberculosis

   C. recurrent epistaxis
   D. status asthmaticus

10. Leukotrienes occur naturally in which of the following?

    A. white blood cells
    B. red blood cells

    C. spermatocytes
    D. none of the above

11. Which of the following agents are used to prevent asthma symptoms?

    A. ephedrine
    B. cromolyn

    C. dextromethorphan
    D. benzonatate

12. Bupropion (Zyban®) is classified as which of the following?

    A. an antiemetic
    B. an anti-asthmatic

    C. an antidepressant
    D. an anticonvulsant

13. All of the following are chronic obstructive pulmonary diseases, except:

    A. emphysema
    B. pneumonia

    C. bronchiectasis
    D. chronic cystic fibrosis

14. Which of the following agents is an expectorant?

    A. guaifenesin (Robitussin®)
    B. hydrocodone (Hycodan®)

    C. oxymetazoline (Afrin®)
    D. nedocromil (Tilade®)

15. Which of the following is the generic name for Singulair®?

    A. zileuton
    B. cromolyn

    C. montelukast
    D. zafirlukast

16. Epinephrine is used for which of the following respiratory disorders?

    A. smoking cessation
    B. chronic cystic fibrosis

    C. temporary relief of nasal congestion
    D. temporary relief of bronchospasm

17. Which of the following agents is a leukotriene modifier?

    A. cromolyn sodium (Intal®)
    B. zafirlukast (Accolate®)

    C. beclomethasone (Vancenase®)
    D. metaproterenol (Alupent®)

18. Which of the following drugs are bronchodilators?

    A. beta-agonists
    B. anticholinergics

    C. methylxanthines
    D. all of the above

19. All of the following are glucocorticoid agents, except:

    A. flunisolide (AeroBid®)
    B. triamcinolone (Azmacort®)

    C. budesonide (Pulmicort®)
    D. pseudoephedrine (Sudafed®)

20. Decongestants are contraindicated in patients with which of the following conditions or disorders?

    A. hypertrophy of the prostate
    B. diabetes mellitus

    C. glaucoma
    D. all of the above

Matching—Terms and Descriptions

Match the lettered term to its numbered description.

Description

_____ 1. An enlargement in the airway at the top of the trachea

_____ 2. Small, microscopic air sacs

_____ 3. The destruction of the alveolar walls

_____ 4. Walls of the bronchioles

_____ 5. Affecting the exocrine glands causing obstruction of the bronchioles

_____ 6. Exposure to a particular antigen

Term

A. Septae

B. Allergy

C. Emphysema

D. Cystic fibrosis

E. Alveoli

F. Larynx

Matching—Drug Names

Match the generic and trade names

Generic Name

_____ 1. ipratropium

_____ 2. bitolterol

_____ 3. metaproterenol

_____ 4. nedocromil

_____ 5. naphazoline

_____ 6. xylometazoline

_____ 7. budesonide

_____ 8. levalbuterol

Trade Name

A. Xopenex®

B. Otrivin®

C. Privine®

D. Pulmicort®

E. Tilade®

F. Tornalate®

G. Alupent®

H. Atrovent®

Fill in the Blank

Select terms from your reading to fill in the blanks.

1. A genetic disorder causing thick mucus to obstruct the bronchioles in the lungs is referred to as _____.

2. The causes of emphysema may include genetics and _____.

3. The neurochemical mechanism of the antidepressant effect of bupropion is _____.

4. Drug administration with a metered dose inhaler (MDI) is often accomplished with one or two _____ from a hand-held pressurized device.

5. Inhaled glucocorticoids are preferred for the long-term control of asthma and are first-line agents for patients with _____ asthma.

6. Quick-relief asthma medicines are also referred to as _____ inhalers.

7. Epinephrine is a naturally occurring catecholamine that may be obtained from animal _____ glands.

8. Xanthine derivatives are also known as _____ and are used to relieve asthma.

9. Bronchodilators are agents that widen the _____ of the _____ tubes.

10. Common adverse effects of H$_1$-receptor antagonists include _____, dizziness, headache, urinary retention, nausea, vomiting, sedation, leukopenia, and _____.

11. Leukotrienes contribute to the inflammation associated with _____.

12. The greatest concentration of histamine is in the skin, _____, and gastrointestinal tract.

13. Lungs are soft, spongy, cone-shaped organs in the _____.

14. Leukotrienes are slow-reacting substances that produce effects similar to those of _____.

15. Theophylline and aminophylline are examples of _____

16. Anti-inflammatory medications for treatment of asthma include glucocorticoids, leukotriene modifiers, and _____ stabilizers.

17. Long-term use of inhaled glucocorticoids in _____ is not recommended because these agents may suppress growth and suppress the _____ glands for production of hormones.

18. Leukotriene antagonists block the bronchoconstriction, mucus production, and _____ that occur with asthma.

19. The main adverse effects of montelukast (Singulair®) are headaches and _____ symptoms.

20. Cromolyn is the drug of choice as a prophylactic for moderate allergic asthma, especially in _____.

True or False

Select the letter "T" or "F" for the following questions.

____ 1. Decongestants cause vasoconstriction of nasal mucosa and reduce swelling.

____ 2. There are specific expectorants indicated for the treatment of tuberculosis.

____ 3. Chronic bronchitis involves significant changes in the bronchi resulting from constant irritation due to smoking or exposure to industrial pollution.

____ 4. The most common uses for decongestants are the relief of headache and glaucoma.

____ 5. Cigarette smoking causes cancers of the pancreas, kidneys, and cervix.

____ 6. Inflammation may result from tissue injury, which damages cells.

____ 7. The chemical mediators that are mostly involved with allergies and asthma include epinephrine and acetylcholine.

____ 8. There are four types of histamines in our body.

____ 9. The nasal mucosa is rich with mast cells.

____ 10. Cigarette smoking can cause the lungs to develop bacterial pneumonia.

ANSWER KEY

Multiple Choice

1. C	2. B	3. D	4. B	5. C
6. B	7. C	8. A	9. D	10. A
11. B	12. C	13. B	14. A	15. C
16. D	17. B	18. D	19. D	20. D

Matching—Terms and Descriptions

1. F	2. E	3. C	4. A	5. D	6. B

Matching—Drug Names

1. H	2. F	3. G	4. E	5. C
6. B	7. D	8. A		

Fill in the Blank

1. cystic fibrosis	2. smoking	3. unknown
4. puffs	5. persistent	6. rescue
7. adrenal	8. bronchodilators	9. diameter; bronchial
10. dry mouth; hypotension	11. asthma	12. lungs
13. thoracic cavity	14. histamine	15. methylxanthines
16. mast cell	17. children; adrenal	18. inflammation
19. GI	20. children	

True or False

1. T	2. F	3. T	4. F	5. T
6. T	7. F	8. F	9. T	10. T

Drug Therapy for Gastrointestinal Disorders

Multiple Choice

Select the correct answer from choices A–D.

1. Mucosal injury in the acid peptic diseases include which of the following?

   A. ulcerative colitis
   B. diverticulitis

   C. disseminated ulcers in the gastrointestinal tract
   D. gastroesophageal reflux disease

2. Histamine antagonists inhibit acid secretion that is stimulated by which of the following chemical substances?

   A. gastrin and acetylcholine
   B. gastrin only

   C. acetylcholine only
   D. bile acid

3. Antibiotics are used to treat peptic ulcers caused by which of the following agents?

   A. E. coli
   B. H. pylori

   C. Salmonella
   D. *Staphylococcus aureus*

4. Antacids neutralize hydrochloric acid and raise gastric pH by which of the following mechanisms?

   A. inhibiting mucus
   B. inhibiting amylase

   C. inhibiting pepsin
   D. inhibiting bile acid

5. Which of the following agents is a proton pump inhibitor?

   A. famotidine
   B. omeprazole

   C. nizatidine
   D. loperamide

6. Which of the following is the generic name for Lomotil®?

   A. bismuth subsalicylate
   B. loperamide

   C. difenoxin with atropine
   D. diphenoxylate with atropine

7. The primary role of antacids in the management of acid-peptic disorders is which of the following?

   A. the cure of ulcers
   B. the relief of pain

   C. the inhibition of ulcers
   D. the prevention of cancers

8. Diarrhea in children may become a medical emergency in as little as 24 hours because of:

   A. the loss of blood
   B. the loss of electrolytes

   C. high fever
   D. abdominal pain

9. Which of the following histamine H_2-receptor antagonists was the first approved for clinical use?

   A. famotidine   C. ranitidine
   B. cimetidine   D. nizatidine

10. Which of the following is the generic name for Tums®?

   A. calcium carbonate with magnesium hydroxide   C. sodium bicarbonate
   B. aluminum hydroxide   D. calcium carbonate

11. Mineral oil is a lubricant laxative that acts in the colon to:

   A. increase water secretion   C. increase electrolyte secretion
   B. increase water retention   D. inhibit blood loss

12. Which of the following antidiarrheals are the most effective drugs for controlling diarrhea?

   A. difenoxin with atropine (Motofen®)   C. bismuth subsalicylate (Pepto-Bismol®)
   B. loperamide (Imodium®)   D. camphorated opium tincture (Paregoric®)

13. Which of the following H_2-receptor agents is the most potent?

   A. ranitidine (Zantac®)   C. famotidine (Pepcid®)
   B. nizatidine (Axid®)   D. cimetidine (Tagamet®)

14. Long-term use of omeprazole (Prilosec®) is contraindicated in patients who:

   A. have gastroesophageal reflux disease   C. are lactating
   B. have duodenal ulcers   D. all of the above

15. Which of the following is a naturally occurring bile acid that is made by the liver and secreted in the bile?

   A. uricosuric   C. urea
   B. ursodiol   D. none of the above

16. Gastric pump inhibitors inhibit hydrogen ions and:

   A. Ca^{++} C. K^+
   B. Na^+ D. Cl^-

17. Which of the following is the generic name for Decadron®?

   A. methylprednisolone   C. dexamethasone
   B. droperidol   D. promethazine

18. Adsorbents are used for which of the following?

   A. chronic constipation   C. acute appendicitis
   B. acute poisoning   D. chronic diverticulitis

19. Which of the following is the generic name for Nexium®?

   A. omeprazole   C. lansoprazole
   B. esomeprazole   D. pantoprazole

20. The newest H_2-receptor antagonist is:

   A. nizatidine   C. famotidine
   B. cimetidine   D. ranitidine

Matching—Drug Names

Match the generic and trade names

Generic Name		Trade Name
_____ 1. aluminum hydroxide		A. Riopan®
_____ 2. glycerin		B. Viokase®
_____ 3. mineral oil		C. Maalox®
_____ 4. pancreatin		D. Prevacid®
_____ 5. bisacodyl		E. Entozyme®
_____ 6. pancrelipase		F. Zofran®
_____ 7. lansoprazole		G. Fleet Babylax®
_____ 8. magnesium hydroxide with aluminum hydroxide		H. Kondremul®
_____ 9. ondansetron		I. Dulcolax®
_____ 10. magaldrate		J. Amphojel®

Fill in the Blank

Select terms from your reading to fill in the blanks.

1. Proton pump inhibitors are widely used in the short-term therapy of _____ and _____ ulcers.

2. Family history, smoking tobacco, and infection with *Helicobacter pylori* may cause _____.

3. The breakdown of large food particles into smaller pieces by physical means is referred to as _____ digestion.

4. The treatment of peptic ulcer includes: antacids, H_2-receptor antagonists, proton pump inhibitors, and _____.

5. Orally administered antacids should be taken 30 to 60 minutes _____ meals.

6. Gastroesophageal reflux disease involves the periodic flow of _____ contents into the _____.

7. *H. pylori* is found in 75 percent of _____ ulcers.

8. Adverse effects of bismuth products include neurotoxicity, dark _____, and dark tongue.

9. The main pancreatic enzymes aid in the digestion of fats, _____, and _____.

10. An emetic is a drug that induces _____.

11. The mechanism of action of antiemetics is largely _____, except that they help to relax the portion of the brain that _____ muscles that cause vomiting.

12. For the eradication of *H. pylori* and healing of duodenal and gastric ulcers via drug therapy, special antibiotics must be added. These antibiotics include amoxicillin, clarithromycin, tetracycline, and _____ (Flagyl®).

13. Syrup of ipecac is the OTC drug used to bring about _____ and should be included in any home emergency kit.

14. Adsorbents should be used cautiously in infants or children younger than _____ years, and in _____ patients.

15. Ursodiol is used to prevent cholesterol _____ from forming during rapid loss of weight.

16. Diphenoxylate (Lomotil®) is a narcotic-related agent that has no _____ activity, but causes sedation and euphoria.

17. Pancrelipase is used as replacement therapy in the symptomatic treatment of _____ syndrome due to cystic fibrosis.

18. Most gallstones are formed from _____.

19. The trade name for sorbitol is _____.

20. The oral preparations of stimulant laxatives usually have an onset of action within _____ hours.

True or False

Select the letter "T" or "F" for the following questions.

____ 1. Adsorbents can inactivate syrup of ipecac and laxatives with activated charcoal.

____ 2. Antidiarrheal agents are used to treat constipation.

____ 3. Peptic ulcer is more common in blood group O.

____ 4. The most widely used antacids are omeprazole and esomeprazole magnesium.

____ 5. Proton pump inhibitors should be taken after meals.

____ 6. Constipation can occur in patients using calcium carbonate and aluminum containing antacids.

____ 7. Softening of the bone is called hyperphosphatemia.

____ 8. The pancreas produces and secretes glucagon.

____ 9. The liver stores glycogen and iron.

____ 10. The large intestine absorbs carbohydrates and vitamins.

ANSWER KEY

Multiple Choice

1. D	2. A	3. B	4. C	5. B
6. D	7. B	8. B	9. B	10. D
11. B	12. D	13. A	14. D	15. B
16. C	17. C	18. B	19. B	20. A

Matching—Drug Names

1. J	2. G	3. H	4. E	5. I
6. B	7. D	8. C	9. F	10. A

Fill in the Blank

1. duodenal; gastric	2. peptic ulcer	3. mechanical
4. antibiotics	5. before	6. gastric; esophagus
7. duodenal	8. stools	9. carbohydrates; proteins
10. vomiting	11. unknown; controls	12. metronidazole
13. vomiting	14. three; elderly	15. gallstones
16. analgesic	17. malabsorption	18. cholesterol
19. Sorbitol	20. 6 to 10	

True or False

1. T	2. F	3. T	4. F	5. F
6. T	7. F	8. T	9. T	10. F

Hormonal Therapy for Endocrine Gland Disorders

Multiple Choice

Select the correct answer from choices A–D.

1. Which of the following hormones stimulates ovarian follicle growth and estrogen secretion?

   A. hypothalamic-releasing hormone
   B. luteinizing hormone
   C. follicle-stimulating hormone
   D. thyroid-stimulating hormone

2. Calcitonin is released by which of the following glands?

   A. pancreas
   B. parathyroid
   C. thyroid
   D. adrenal cortex

3. Which of the following hormones maintains the level of glucose in the blood through glycogenolysis?

   A. insulin
   B. glucagon
   C. aldosterone
   D. oxytocin

4. Radioactive iodine is used in which of the following disorders or conditions?

   A. hypothyroidism
   B. hyperthyroidism
   C. thyroiditis
   D. all of the above

5. Which of the following is the mechanism of action of propylthiouracil?

   A. totally inhibiting the peripheral conversion of T_4 to T_3
   B. partially inhibiting the peripheral conversion of T_4 to T_3
   C. totally inhibiting the peripheral conversion of T_3 to T_4
   D. partially inhibiting the peripheral conversion of T_3 to T_4

6. Which of the following conditions is a form of hyperadrenalism?

   A. Cushing's syndrome
   B. Conn's syndrome
   C. Addison's disease
   D. A and B

7. Regular insulin is also available as:

   A. Humulin® 70/30
   B. Novolin® N 80/20
   C. Humulin® 50/50
   D. A and C

8. Diabetes insipidus results from a deficiency of:

   A. PRL
   B. ACTH
   C. ADH
   D. PTH

9. The primary effects of aldosterone include which of the following statements?

    A. It increases water and sodium kidney reabsorption.
    B. It increases blood calcium levels by stimulating bone demineralization.
    C. It increases kidney reabsorption of calcium and potassium.
    D. all of the above

10. The adrenal medulla secretes which of the following hormones?

    A. calcitonin
    B. cortisol
    C. oxytocin
    D. epinephrine

11. Which of the following hormones produces milk?

    A. calcitonin
    B. prolactin
    C. oxytocin
    D. cortisol

12. Growth hormone is secreted by:

    A. the hypothalamus
    B. the anterior pituitary gland
    C. the posterior pituitary gland
    D. all of the above

13. Methimazole is classified as which of the following agents?

    A. an antiemetic
    B. an antithyroid agent
    C. an antipsychotic
    D. an antiestrogen

14. Which of the following is the treatment of hypothyroidism?

    A. estrogen and vitamin C
    B. thyroid hormone and vitamin D
    C. thyroid hormone and calcitonin
    D. calcium salts and vitamin D

15. Prolonged use of glucocorticoids may suppress which of the following endocrine glands?

    A. pancreas
    B. pituitary
    C. pineal
    D. all of the above

16. Humulin 70/30 is a mixture of:

    A. 70 percent insulin zinc and 30 percent regular insulin
    B. 70 percent isophane insulin and 30 percent regular insulin
    C. 70 percent regular insulin and 30 percent isophane insulin
    D. 70 percent regular insulin and 30 percent insulin zinc

17. Which of the following is the generic name for Glucophage®?

    A. repaglinide
    B. acarbose
    C. glipizide
    D. metformin

18. Norepinephrine is released from the medulla of the adrenal glands, and mineralocorticoids are released from the:

    A. thyroid
    B. adrenal cortex
    C. breast
    D. pituitary

19. Adrenocorticotropic hormone (ACTH) primarily stimulates secretion of which of the following hormones?

    A. estrogen
    B. cortisol
    C. testosterone
    D. insulin

20. Luteinizing hormone is secreted by which of the following glands?

    A. ovaries
    B. testes
    C. both ovaries and testes
    D. none of the above

Matching—Terms and Descriptions

Match the lettered term to its numbered description.

Description	Term
1. _____ The ends of long bones that are originally separated from the main bone by a layer of cartilage	A. Dwarfism
2. _____ An autoimmune disorder of the thyroid gland	B. Gigantism
3. _____ Overdevelopment of the bones of the head, face, and feet	C. Hirsuitism
4. _____ A condition of thyroid insufficiency	D. Acromegaly
5. _____ A condition of lack of growth of the arms and legs in proportion to the head and trunk	E. Myxedema
6. _____ A condition that produces excessive growth prior to puberty	F. Tremors
7. _____ Involuntary trembling (rhythmic shaking) that affects either the limbs or the trunk	G. Epiphyses
8. _____ Excessive hair growth on the face, abdomen, chest, and back	H. Graves' disease

Fill in the Blank

Select terms from your reading to fill in the blanks.

1. Prolactin is a hormone that is primarily associated with _____.

2. The process by which male gametes develop into mature spermatozoa is called _____.

3. Neural pathways connect the hypothalamus to the _____ pituitary gland.

4. Hormones are secreted primarily via the urine and, to a lesser extent, via the _____.

5. Growth hormone is prescribed for _____.

6. In females, an acute rise of LH triggers _____.

7. Thyroxine is the major hormone secreted by the follicular cells of the _____ gland.

8. Calcitonin participates in calcium and _____ metabolism.

9. The release of glucagon prevents the development of _____.

10. The main indication for replacement of growth hormone is growth failure in _____.

11. Long-term use of thyroxine may cause _____.

12. Addison's disease results when the adrenal glands fail to produce corticosteroids and _____.

13. The trade name of cortisone acetate is _____.

14. Insulin-dependent diabetes mellitus is type _____.

15. A patient's body in diabetes mellitus type 1 tends to be _____, while in diabetes mellitus type 2 it tends to be _____.

16. Oral hypoglycemic agents stimulate the pancreas to secrete more _____ and increase the sensitivity of insulin receptors in _____ tissues.

17. Adrenogenital syndrome is a group of disorders involving _____ hormone production in the adrenal glands.

18. Epinephrine (adrenaline) is produced by the medulla of the _____ glands, and is a "fight or flight" hormone that is released when danger threatens.

19. Mineralocorticoids are steroid hormones that influence _____ and _____ balance; they are released from the adrenal cortex.

20. Endocrine glands secrete _____, or chemical messengers, directly into the _____.

True or False

Select the letter "T" or "F" for the following questions.

____ 1. The major hormone secreted by the follicular cells of the thyroid gland is oxytocin.

____ 2. Luteinizing hormone in women stimulates ovum maturation and ovulation.

____ 3. Hypothalamic-releasing hormones stimulate the posterior pituitary to secrete oxytocin.

____ 4. Alpha-cells of the pancreas secrete insulin.

____ 5. The majority of hormones such as thyroxine, insulin, and growth hormone are steroids.

____ 6. ACTH is used generally for diagnostic testing, and not for therapeutic purposes.

____ 7. In males, LH is also called "Interstitial Cell Stimulating Hormone" because it stimulates the production of testosterone.

____ 8. Calcitonin is produced primarily by the parafollicular cells of the thyroid gland.

____ 9. Diabetes insipidus is a disease that results from a deficiency of insulin.

____ 10. Graves' disease is an example of hypothyroidism and it is far more common in men than in women.

ANSWER KEY

Multiple Choice

1. C	2. C	3. B	4. B	5. B
6. D	7. D	8. C	9. A	10. D
11. B	12. B	13. B	14. D	15. B
16. B	17. D	18. B	19. B	20. D

Matching—Terms and Descriptions

1. G	2. H	3. D	4. E	5. A
6. B	7. F	8. C		

Fill in the Blank

1. lactation	2. spermatogenesis	3. posterior
4. bile	5. dwarfism	6. ovulation
7. thyroid	8. phosphorus	9. hypoglycemia
10. children	11. osteoporosis	12. aldosterone
13. Cortone®	14. I	15. thin; obese
16. insulin; target	17. steroid	18. adrenal
19. salt; water	20. hormones; bloodstream	

True or False

1. F	2. T	3. F	4. F	5. F
6. T	7. T	8. T	9. F	10. F

CHAPTER 17

Hormones of the Reproductive System and Contraceptives

Multiple Choice

Select the correct answer from choices A–D.

1. Naturally occurring estrogens include which of the following?

   A. estradiol
   B. estriol
   C. estrone
   D. all of the above

2. One of the most common adverse effects of estrogens is:

   A. primary ovarian failure
   B. thromboembolic disorders
   C. amenorrhea
   D. hypogonadism

3. Progesterone is secreted primarily by which of the following?

   A. hypothalamus
   B. pituitary
   C. adrenal medulla
   D. ovaries

4. Progesterone is indicated in which of the following cases?

   A. habitual abortion
   B. infertility
   C. irregular uterine bleeding
   D. all of the above

5. All of the following are androgens, except:

   A. testosterone enanthate (Delatest®)
   B. finasteride (Proscar®)
   C. fluoxymesterone (Halotestin®)
   D. methyltestosterone (Android®)

6. Which of the following is an anabolic steroid?

   A. stanozolol (Winstrol®)
   B. finasteride (Proscar)
   C. norgestrel (Ovrette®)
   D. norethindrone (Norlutin®)

7. Oxytocic agents are used to initiate or improve:

   A. uterine relaxation only after the cervix is dilated
   B. uterine contraction at term only in carefully selected patients
   C. both A and B
   D. none of the above

8. Which of the following microorganisms may cause genital warts?

   A. chlamydia trachomatis
   B. herpes simplex 1

   C. herpes simplex 2
   D. human papillomavirus

9. Which of the following is the indication of testosterone?

   A. cryptorchidism
   B. prostate cancer

   C. breast cancer in men
   D. prostatic hyperplasia

10. Which of the following is the mechanism of action of anabolic steroids?

    A. They change the uterine lining from a proliferative structure to a secretory one.
    B. They promote tissue building processes.

    C. They bind to extracellular receptors that stimulate RNA and DNA to synthesize proteins responsible for the effects of testosterone.
    D. none of the above

11. Absence of blood flow during menstruation is referred to as:

    A. menorrhagia
    B. metrorrhagia

    C. amenorrhea
    D. none of the above

12. Progesterone is contraindicated in patients with:

    A. undiagnosed vaginal bleeding
    B. thrombophlebitis

    C. breast cancer
    D. all of the above

13. Uterine stimulant agents cause contractions of the myometrium during:

    A. labor and delivery
    B. menses

    C. menopause
    D. all of the above

14. Penicillin G is the drug of choice for which of the following sexually transmitted diseases?

    A. genital warts
    B. genital herpes

    C. syphilis
    D. chlamydia

15. Metronidazole should be prescribed for which of the following sexually transmitted diseases?

    A. trichomoniasis
    B. gonorrhea

    C. syphilis
    D. chlamydia

16. Which of the following drugs is an androgen?

    A. testosterone
    B. norethindrone

    C. androsterone
    D. A and C

17. Which of the following is the generic name for Depo-Provera®?

    A. norethindrone
    B. medroxyprogesterone

    C. norgestrel
    D. none of the above

18. Uterine relaxants are contraindicated in patients with which of the following conditions?

    A. pneumonia
    B. antepartum hemorrhage

    C. eclampsia
    D. B and C

19. Estrogens are contraindicated in which of the following?

    A. undiagnosed abnormal uterine bleeding
    B. ovarian failure

    C. prostate cancer
    D. amenorrhea

20. Which of the following is the mechanism of action of fixed combinations of estrogen and progestin?

    A. They prevent maturation of sperm.
    B. They prevent ovulation and sperm penetration.

    C. They prevent the ovaries from releasing eggs.
    D. none of the above

Matching—Terms and Descriptions

Match the lettered term to its numbered description.

Description	Term
1. _____ Pathway of sperm to exit the testes	A. Uterus
2. _____ Manufactures estrogen	B. Penis
3. _____ Houses the growing embryo	C. Testes
4. _____ Transports sperm to female reproductive system	D. Ovary
5. _____ Pathway through which the egg moves to the uterus	E. Fallopian tube
6. _____ Manufacture testosterone	F. Seminal duct

Matching—Drug Names

Match the generic and trade names.

Generic Name	Trade Name
1. _____ progesterone	A. Norlutin®
2. _____ oxandrolone	B. Winstrol®
3. _____ fluoxymesterone	C. Delatest®
4. _____ stanozolol	D. Premarin®
5. _____ finasteride	E. Proscar®
6. _____ conjugated estrogen	F. Oxandrin®
7. _____ norethindrone	G. Halotestin®
8. _____ testosterone enanthate	H. Gesterol®

Fill in the Blank

Select terms from your reading to fill in the blanks.

1. The most important androgenic hormone produced by the _____ in males is _____.

2. Oral contraceptives are hormone medications for the prevention of _____.

3. The natural estrogens may be administered by the intramuscular or _____ route.

4. FSH is secreted by the _____.

5. An oral contraceptive is commonly referred to as the "_____."

6. Progesterone in high doses suppresses the pituitary's release of _____.

7. Generally, two types of medications are used during labor and delivery: uterine stimulants and _____.

8. Anabolic steroids are similar to _____.

9. The natural estrogens, such as ethinyl estradiol, may be administered _____.

10. Gonadotropin-releasing hormone stimulates the release of _____ and _____ from the anterior pituitary gland.

11. Testosterone stimulates the development of the male _____ sex characteristics and initiates the production of _____.

12. The corpus luteum secretes _____ only during the _____ two weeks of the menstrual cycle.

13. _____ is used in the treatment of endometriosis and premenstrual syndrome.

14. The use of estrogen-progestin combinations in a cyclic fashion generally results in the inhibition of _____ without preventing menstruation.

15. Depot-medroxyprogesterone acetate (Depo-Provera®) is a long-acting _____.

16. The greatest amount of progesterone is secreted during the week after _____ has taken place.

17. Contraceptives are contraindicated in _____ (category X), lactation, and missed abortion.

18. Oxytocic agents promote the _____ reflex in nursing mothers.

19. Progesterone causes an increase in the viscosity of _____ secretions.

20. Two agents are currently used as uterine relaxants: ritodrine (Yutopar®) and terbutaline (_____).

True or False

Select the letter "T" or "F" for the following questions.

____ 1. The male reproductive system is composed of two testes and two fallopian tubes.

____ 2. FSH is secreted by the ovaries and testes.

____ 3. The ovaries and testes inhibit secretion of LH from the pituitary by negative feedback.

____ 4. The most common adverse effects of estrogens are breast swelling, weight gain, and hypertension.

____ 5. The trade name of ethinyl estradiol is Feminone®.

____ 6. A blood clot in the bloodstream is called "arteriosclerosis."

____ 7. Uterine relaxants often alter fetal and maternal heart rates and maternal blood pressure.

____ 8. Gonorrhea is caused by the human papillomavirus.

____ 9. Androgens are secreted mainly in the interstitial tissue of the testes.

____ 10. Androgen hormone inhibitors such as finasteride (Proscar®) are used in the treatment of benign tumor of the female breast.

ANSWER KEY

Multiple Choice

1. D	2. B	3. D	4. D	5. B
6. A	7. B	8. D	9. A	10. B
11. C	12. D	13. A	14. C	15. A
16. D	17. B	18. D	19. A	20. B

Matching—Terms and Descriptions

1. F	2. D	3. A	4. B	5. E	6. C

Matching—Drug Names

1. H	2. F	3. G	4. B	5. E
6. D	7. A	8. C		

Fill in the Blank

1. testes; testosterone	2. pregnancy	3. subcutaneous
4. pituitary	5. pill	6. LH
7. uterine relaxants	8. androgens	9. orally
10. FSH; LH	11. secondary; sperm	12. last
13. Progesterone	14. conception	15. progestin
16. ovulation	17. pregnancy	18. milk ejection
19. cervical	20. Brethine®	

True or False

1. F	2. F	3. T	4. T	5. T
6. F	7. T	8. F	9. T	10. F

CHAPTER 18

Diuretics

Multiple Choice

Select the correct answer from choices A–D.

1. Which of the following terms means "inability to produce urine"?

   A. disuria
   B. polyuria

   C. anuria
   D. uremia

2. Having a lower osmotic pressure than a reference solution is referred to as:

   A. hypotonic
   B. hypertonic

   C. isotonic
   D. none of the above

3. Which of the following sites is where the process of filtration occurs?

   A. the loop of Henle
   B. the renal corpuscle

   C. the distal convoluted tubule
   D. the collecting tubule

4. Which of the following parts of the urinary system stores urine?

   A. renal pelvis
   B. renal calyces

   C. renal tubule
   D. urinary bladder

5. Diuretic drugs are an important part of management of:

   A. weight gain
   B. hypotension

   C. heart failure
   D. gallbladder stones

6. All of the following are categories of diuretic drugs, except:

   A. potassium-sparing
   B. alpha and beta blockers

   C. loop diuretics
   D. carbonic anhydrase inhibitors

7. Which of the following is the generic name of Demadex®?

   A. torsemide
   B. furosemide

   C. bumetanide
   D. ethacrynic acid

8. Which of the following agents are the most efficacious and rapidly absorbed type of diuretics?

   A. loop diuretics
   B. thiazide-like diuretics

   C. osmotic diuretics
   D. potassium-sparing diuretics

9. Which of the following diuretics are still considered to be in the front line for the treatment of mild to moderate hypertension, either on their own or combined?

   A. carbonic anhydrase inhibitors
   B. potassium-sparing diuretics

   C. thiazide diuretics
   D. loop diuretics

10. Thiazide diuretics are contraindicated in which of the following patients?

    A. those with electrolyte imbalances
    B. those in hepatic coma
    C. those with anuria
    D. all of the above

11. All of the following are classified as potassium-sparing diuretics, except:

    A. mannitol (Osmitrol®)
    B. triamterene (Dyrenium®)
    C. amiloride (Midamor®)
    D. spironolactone (Aldactone®)

12. Osmotic diuretics should be avoided in patients with which of the following conditions or disorders?

    A. known hypersensitivity
    B. intracranial pressure
    C. intracranial bleeding
    D. history of gout

13. Which of the following is the generic name for Osmoglyn®?

    A. mannitol
    B. chlorthalidone
    C. polythiazide
    D. glycerin

14. Loop diuretics (such as furosemide) are used for which of the following?

    A. the management of severe chronic heart failure
    B. the treatment of acute heart failure
    C. severe electrolyte deficiency
    D. both A and B

15. When a patient is taking carbonic anhydrase inhibitors, which of the following should be monitored?

    A. fluid output
    B. electrolyte levels
    C. glucose levels
    D. all of the above

16. Approximately how much urine is formed per minute in the kidneys?

    A. 1 mL
    B. 10 mL
    C. 25 mL
    D. 125 mL

17. Which of the following is the generic name for Mykrox®?

    A. urea
    B. mannitol
    C. metolazone
    D. glycerin

18. Which of the following are the adverse effects of carbonic anhydrase inhibitors?

    A. renal stones and acidosis
    B. hyperkalemia
    C. respiratory alkalosis
    D. metabolic alkalosis

19. Which of the following is the mechanism of action for potassium-sparing diuretics?

    A. They inhibit the reabsorption of chloride and calcium.
    B. They inhibit the action of carbonic anhydrase.
    C. They inhibit the action of aldosterone in the nephrons.
    D. They increase reabsorption of sodium and potassium.

20. Spironolactone has proved to be of tremendous value in the treatment of:

    A. chronic bronchitis
    B. congestive heart failure
    C. hyperkalemia
    D. hyponatremia

Matching—Terms and Descriptions

Match the lettered term to its numbered description.

Description	Term
1. _____ Low blood level of potassium	A. Glomerulus
2. _____ Enlargement of breast tissue in males	B. Impotence
3. _____ Low blood level of sodium	C. Hypokalemia
4. _____ Inability to produce urine	D. Anuria
5. _____ Inability to achieve penile erection	E. Hyponatremia
6. _____ A set of capillary loops	F. Gynecomastia

Matching—Drug Names

Match the generic and trade names.

Generic Name	Trade Name
1. _____ bumetanide	A. Diuril®
2. _____ hydrochlorothiazide	B. Oratrol®
3. _____ amiloride hydrochloride	C. Dyrenium®
4. _____ torsemide	D. Neptazane®
5. _____ dichlorphenamide	E. Bumex®
6. _____ methazolamide	F. Demadex®
7. _____ triamterene	G. HCTZ®
8. _____ chlorothiazide sodium	H. Midamor®

Fill in the Blank

Select terms from your reading to fill in the blanks.

1. The urinary system functions to remove _____ materials from the _____ tissues and fluids.

2. The kidneys consist of two distinct regions: inner (medulla) and outer (_____).

3. The urinary bladder is within the _____ cavity.

4. Diuretics are divided into _____ categories according to their action.

5. Antidiuretic hormone is released from the _____ gland.

6. Having a lower osmotic pressure than water is referred to as _____.

7. A major problem of loop diuretics is the loss of _____ from the body.

8. Thiazide drugs act on the cortical segment of the _____ loop and _____ convoluted tubules of the nephron.

9. Thiazide can cause _____, which is potentially dangerous in diabetics.

10. The best-known aldosterone antagonist is _____.

11. Osmotic diuretics work by directly interfering with _____.

12. Thiazide diuretics should be given with caution during pregnancy and lactation, in children, and with _____ or _____ impairment.

13. The optimum therapeutic effects of thiazides are seen in 15 to 30 minutes when given _____.

14. Uric acid levels may rise during _____ diuretic therapy, which can be problematic for people with gout.

15. Adverse effects of osmotic diuretics include electrolyte imbalance and the potential for _____.

16. The kidneys are connected to the urinary bladder by _____.

17. The urinary system helps maintain _____ by regulating the composition, volume, and pH of extracellular fluid.

18. The major calyces empty urine into the _____.

19. The internal floor of the urinary bladder includes a triangular area called the _____.

20. Osmotic diuretics should be used with caution in patients with electrolyte imbalances or _____ impairment.

True or False

Select the letter "T" or "F" for the following questions.

____ 1. Diuretics are mainly used to treat edema.

____ 2. The structures of the urinary system include two kidneys and two urethra.

____ 3. The urinary bladder is the basic structural unit of the kidney.

____ 4. The type of diuretic used is determined by the condition being treated.

____ 5. A diuretic compound, such as acetazolamide (Diamox®), is used to lower blood pressure.

____ 6. *Hyperkalemia* is the term used to refer to low levels of sodium in the blood.

____ 7. Thiazide diuretics are contraindicated in patients with unknown hypersensitivity to these agents.

____ 8. Spironolactone has a rather slow onset of action, requiring several days before full therapeutic effects are achieved.

____ 9. Osmotic diuretics can be used to maintain urine volume and to prevent anuria.

____ 10. Carbonic anhydrase is an enzyme that slows down the conversion of carbon dioxide into bicarbonate ions.

ANSWER KEY

Multiple Choice

1. C	2. A	3. B	4. D	5. C
6. B	7. A	8. A	9. C	10. D
11. A	12. C	13. D	14. D	15. D
16. A	17. C	18. A	19. C	20. B

Matching—Terms and Descriptions

1. C	2. F	3. E	4. D	5. B	6. A

Matching—Drug Names

1. E	2. G	3. H	4. F	5. B
6. D	7. C	8. A		

Fill in the Blank

1. waste; body	2. cortex	3. pelvic
4. five	5. pituitary	6. hypotonic
7. electrolytes	8. ascending; distal	9. hyperglycemia
10. spironolactone	11. osmosis	12. liver; kidney
13. intravenously	14. loop	15. dehydration
16. ureters	17. homeostasis	18. renal pelvis
19. trigone	20. renal	

True or False

1. T	2. F	3. F	4. T	5. F
6. F	7. F	8. T	9. T	10. F

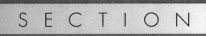

Pharmacology for Disorders Affecting Multi-Body Systems

Vitamins, Minerals, and Nutritional Supplements

Multiple Choice

Select the correct answer from choices A–D.

1. Which of the following vitamin deficiencies may cause rickets?

   A. vitamin C
   B. vitamin A

   C. vitamin D
   D. vitamin K

2. Which of the following signs or symptoms indicates vitamin A toxicity?

   A. hepatotoxicity
   B. hyperlipidemia

   C. hypercalcemia
   D. all of the above

3. Vitamin E is essential for which of the following?

   A. muscle development
   B. normal reproduction

   C. resistance of erythrocytes to hemolysis
   D. all of the above

4. Vitamin K_1 is also referred to as:

   A. phylloquinone
   B. tocopherol

   C. retinol
   D. calciferol

5. Which of the following is the major electrolyte in intracellular fluids?

   A. sodium
   B. potassium

   C. magnesium
   D. chloride

6. Which of the following is a trace element?

   A. phosphorus
   B. calcium

   C. sodium
   D. iron

7. Magnesium is an important ion for the function of:

   A. many enzyme systems
   B. glycogen formation

   C. acid-base balance
   D. hemoglobin formation

8. Vitamin A deficiency leads to which of the following?

   A. muscle degeneration
   B. growth retardation

   C. night blindness
   D. bone loss

9. Deficiency of vitamin B_1 (thiamine) leads to the disease called:

   A. marasmus
   B. rickets

   C. beriberi
   D. osteomalacia

10. Pellagra is characterized by which of the following signs or symptoms?

    A. loss of memory
    B. diarrhea

    C. skin lesions
    D. all of the above

11. Vitamin C is essential for the formation of:

    A. the brain and eye color
    B. eggs in females

    C. bone, cartilage, and skin
    D. the lungs

12. Too much calcium will lead to which of the following conditions?

    A. osteoporosis
    B. cardiac failure

    C. diarrhea
    D. tetany

13. Which of the following microminerals may cause mottling of the teeth?

    A. iodine (I)
    B. copper (Cu)

    C. zinc (Zn)
    D. fluoride (F)

14. Which of the following types of nutritional care is used to meet the patient's nutritional requirements?

    A. enteral nutrition
    B. hyperalimentation

    C. both A and B
    D. none of the above

15. Which of the following vitamin deficiencies may cause spina bifida in a fetus?

    A. vitamin C
    B. vitamin D

    C. vitamin K
    D. folic acid

16. Which of the following may result from phosphorus deficiency?

    A. marasmus
    B. pellagra

    C. pernicious anemia
    D. none of the above

17. Potassium deficiency can cause:

    A. dysrhythmias
    B. constipation

    C. anemia
    D. kidney stones

18. Moderately high amounts of iodine in the diet can be bad for which of the following?

    A. hearing
    B. acne

    C. anemia
    D. vision

19. Thiamin (vitamin B_1) toxicity can result in:

    A. blindness
    B. dysrhythmia

    C. nephrotoxicity
    D. hepatotoxicity

20. Which of the following vitamin deficiencies produces fissures on the lips (cheilosis)?

    A. pyridoxine (vitamin B_6)
    B. hydroxocobalamin (vitamin B_{12})

    C. riboflavin (vitamin B_2)
    D. ascorbic acid (vitamin C)

Matching—Terms and Descriptions

Match the lettered term to its numbered description.

Description   **Term**

1. _____ Fissures on the lips   A. Cachexia

2. _____ Softening, ulceration, and perforation of the cornea   B. Ataxia

3. _____ Weight loss, wasting of muscle, and loss of appetite   C. Hemolysis

4. _____ Destruction of red blood cells and release of hemoglobin   D. Osteomalacia

5. _____ Bone softens and becomes brittle   E. Keratomalacia

6. _____ Loss of the ability to coordinate muscular movement   F. Cheilosis

Matching—Vitamins, Minerals, and Other Elements

Match the lettered term to its numbered description.

Description   **Term**

1. _____ A fat-soluble vitamin   A. Fluorine

2. _____ The major electrolyte in intracellular fluids   B. Copper

3. _____ An essential element for thyroid hormone   C. Phosphorus

4. _____ The major electrolyte in extracellular fluids   D. Iodine

5. _____ A component of DNA and RNA, and essential for all living cells   E. Potassium

6. _____ An essential element for the formation of hemoglobin and myoglobin   F. Sodium

7. _____ Important for the formation of hemoglobin because it is part of   G. Iron
           a co-enzyme

                                                                                 H. Tocopherol
8. _____ Found in shellfish, kelp, and tea

Fill in the Blank

Select terms from your reading to fill in the blanks.

1. An abnormally low level of magnesium in the blood is referred to as _____.

2. Nicotinic acid is also known as vitamin _____ or niacin.

3. Intrinsic factor is secreted by the _____ mucous membranes and is essential for the absorption of vitamin B_{12} in the _____.

4. Any substance that becomes part of a food product is called a _____.

5. Xerophthalmia is an extreme dryness of the _____ of the eyes.

6. Retinol is a fat-soluble vitamin and also known as _____.

7. Vitamin K is essential for the synthesis of prothrombin in the _____.

8. Retinol is not found in plant products, but fortunately, most plants contain substances called _____.

9. Deficiency of vitamin E is _____.

10. In healthy adults, primary vitamin K deficiency is _____.

11. Thiamin (also spelled "thiamine") plays a key role in the metabolic breakdown of _____.

12. Vitamin B_2 (riboflavin) plays an important role in preventing some visual disorders, especially _____.

13. Vitamin B_7 is also known as _____.

14. Vitamin C deficiency causes _____.

15. Pharma food is a system of receiving nourishment through _____.

16. Total parenteral nutrition is used to meet the patient's nutritional requirements when the _____ route cannot accomplish this.

17. The setting of standards and enforcement for nutrition labeling are responsibilities of the _____.

18. Labeling of foods and supplements must be _____ and not misleading.

19. Copper toxicity may be seen in patients with _____ disease.

20. Megadoses of zinc can result in acute toxicity and can be _____.

True or False

Select the letter "T" or "F" for the following questions.

____ 1. Copper, like iron, is important for the synthesis of hemoglobin.

____ 2. Zinc deficiency is characterized by poor appetite and retardation of growth.

____ 3. Radioisotopes of iodine are used in cheilosis.

____ 4. Inorganic substances occurring naturally in the earth's crust are called vitamins.

____ 5. Folic acid is also known as vitamin B_{12}.

____ 6. Sulfur is necessary to all body tissues and is found in all body cells.

____ 7. Insufficient exposure to sunlight and vitamin D may result in cardiovascular disorders.

____ 8. Vitamins A and K are fat-soluble.

____ 9. Vitamin D deficiency may cause keratomalacia.

____ 10. Vitamin B_{12} deficiency causes pernicious anemia and neurological disorders.

ANSWER KEY

Multiple Choice

1. C	2. D	3. D	4. A	5. B
6. D	7. A	8. D	9. C	10. D
11. C	12. B	13. D	14. C	15. D
16. D	17. A	18. B	19. D	20. C

Matching—Terms and Descriptions

1. F	2. E	3. A	4. C	5. D	6. B

Matching—Vitamins, Minerals, and Other Elements

1. H	2. E	3. D	4. F	5. C
6. G	7. B	8. A		

Fill in the Blank

1. hypomagnesemia	2. B_3	3. gastric; intestines
4. food additive	5. conjunctiva	6. vitamin A
7. liver	8. carotenoids	9. rare
10. uncommon	11. carbohydrates	12. cataracts
13. biotin	14. scurvy	15. breathing
16. enteral	17. FDA	18. accurate
19. Wilson's	20. fatal	

True or False

1. T	2. T	3. F	4. F	5. F
6. T	7. F	8. T	9. F	10. T

CHAPTER 20

Antineoplastic Agents

Multiple Choice

Select the correct answer from choices A–D.

1. Which of the following is/are the main pathway(s) of spreading malignant tumor cells?

   A. via the blood
   B. through the lymphocytes

   C. by seeding the surface of the body cavities
   D. all of the above

2. The cause of most human cancers is:

   A. sunlight (UV radiation)
   B. cigarette smoking

   C. radiation
   D. unknown

3. Anticancer drugs may be given to attempt a cure for which of the following purposes?

   A. to relieve or reduce intensity of uncomfortable symptoms
   B. to prevent cancer from occurring

   C. both A and B
   D. none of the above

4. Which of the following is classified as an antimetabolite?

   A. mercaptopurine (Purinethol®)
   B. flutamide (Eulexin®)

   C. ethinyl acetate (Femring®)
   D. all of the above

5. The mechanism of action of antitumor antibiotics is:

   A. the inhibition of DNA synthesis
   B. the inhibition of RNA synthesis

   C. the inhibition of DNA and RNA synthesis
   D. none of the above

6. Which of the following antitumor antibiotics are used only for the treatment of testicular cancer?

   A. idarubicin (Idamycin PFS®)
   B. plicamycin (Mithramycin®)

   C. dactinomycin (Actinomycin D®)
   D. bleomycin (Blenoxane®)

7. Which of the following classes of antineoplastic agents was the first to be used?

   A. mitotic inhibitors (plant alkaloids)
   B. special antibiotics

   C. alkylating agents
   D. antimetabolites

8. Which of the following is the generic name for Leukeran®?

   A. chlorambucil
   B. carmustine

   C. busulfan
   D. cisplatin

9. Which of the following is the newest type of alkylating agents?

   A. busulfans
   B. temozolomides

   C. nitrosoureas
   D. thiotepas

10. Which of the following antitumor antibiotics are only used for acute leukemia (cancer of the blood)?

    A. idarubicin (Idamycin PFS®)
    B. plicamycin (Mithramycin®)
    C. dactinomycin (Actinomycin D®)
    D. bleomycin (Blenoxane®)

11. Mitotic inhibitors are contraindicated in patients with which of the following?

    A. heart attack or viral infection
    B. leukopenia or bacterial infection
    C. breast cancer or Hodgkin's disease
    D. lymphocytic lymphoma or testicular cancer

12. Which of the following is the major adverse effect of hormonal agents in female patients?

    A. feminization
    B. masculization
    C. bone marrow depression
    D. hepatic and renal toxicity

13. Alkylating agents are used to treat which of the following malignant neoplasms?

    A. brain tumor
    B. Hodgkin's disease
    C. metastatic bladder cancer
    D. all of the above

14. Which of the following are the common adverse effects of antitumor antibiotics?

    A. hair loss
    B. herpes zoster
    C. hyperthermia
    D. bone marrow suppression

15. Which of the following is an indication of vincristine (a mitotic inhibitor drug)?

    A. mental depression
    B. acute leukemia
    C. alopecia
    D. gout

16. Which of the following is the generic name for Thioplex®?

    A. oxaliplatin
    B. cisplatin
    C. busulfan
    D. thiotepa

17. Which of the following is an example of a folic acid antagonist?

    A. mercaptopurine
    B. methotrexate
    C. fluorouracil
    D. none of the above

18. Which of the following is an example of a purine analog?

    A. fluorouracil
    B. methotrexate
    C. mercaptopurine
    D. tamoxifen citrate

19. Antitumor antibiotics are very effective in the treatment of which of the following disorders?

    A. certain malignant tumors
    B. certain benign tumors
    C. acute bacterial infections
    D. chronic bacterial infections

20. Mitotic inhibitors are derived from:

    A. animals
    B. plants
    C. minerals
    D. fat-soluble vitamins

Matching—Terms and Descriptions

Match the lettered term to its numbered description.

Description	Term
1. _____ Any agent directly involved in or related to the promotion of cancer	A. Benign
2. _____ Reducing intensity of uncomfortable symptoms	B. Alopecia
3. _____ Cellular growth that becomes progressively worse	C. Metastasize
4. _____ Spreading from one point of the body to another	D. Malignant
5. _____ Cellular growth that is nonprogressive	E. Palliation
6. _____ Loss of hair from anywhere on the body	F. Carcinogen

Matching—Drug Names

Match the generic and trade names.

Generic Name	Trade Name
1. _____ oxaliplatin	A. Platinol®
2. _____ floxuridine	B. Temodar®
3. _____ pentostatin	C. Valstar®
4. _____ daunorubicin	D. Ellence®
5. _____ cisplatin	E. FUDR®
6. _____ epirubicin	F. Cerubidine®
7. _____ valrubicin	G. Nipent®
8. _____ temozolomide	H. Eloxatin®

Fill in the Blank

Select terms from your reading to fill in the blanks.

1. Only malignant tumor cells have the capacity to _____.

2. The terms *neoplasm* and _____ are used synonymously.

3. The cell cycle may last from 24 hours to _____.

4. Cancer may be treated by using surgery, radiation therapy, and _____.

5. Many malignant lesions are _____ if detected in the early stage.

6. Chemotherapy is often combined with surgery and _____ to increase the probability of a cure.

7. Antimetabolites interfere with the activity of enzymes and alter the _____ structure.

8. A decrease in the number of white blood cells is referred to as _____.

9. The precise action of hormones on malignant neoplasms is _____.

10. Steroids are especially useful in treating lymphomas, _____, and Hodgkin's disease.

11. The major adverse effect of hormonal agents in male patients is _____.

12. The most serious adverse effects of antitumor antibiotics are low blood cell counts and _____ failure.

13. During World War I, chemical warfare was introduced using _____.

14. The newer types of alkylating agents, such as nitrosoureas, are lipid-soluble drugs used in treating brain tumors and testicular or _____ cancers.

15. Vincristine sulfate is classified as a _____ inhibitor, used in acute leukemia.

16. The four phases of the cell cycle consist of a first growth phase (G_1), synthesis (S_1), a second growth phase (G_2) and _____.

17. The classes of antimetabolites include folic acid antagonists, pyrimidine analogs, and _____ analogs.

18. _____ is effective in the treatment of gestational choriocarcinoma and hydatidiform mole.

19. Abarelix, flutamide, and tamoxifen citrates are _____ antagonists.

20. The trade name of vinblastine sulfate is _____.

True or False

Select the letter "T" or "F" for the following questions.

____ 1. The mitosis (M) phase of cell division normally takes 10 hours.

____ 2. Many carcinogens may cause bacterial infections.

____ 3. Methotrexate is also used for acute and subacute endocarditis.

____ 4. Alcohol may enhance CNS depression if taken with antimetabolites.

____ 5. Estrogen may also be administered to postmenopausal women with breast cancer.

____ 6. Major adverse effects of hormonal agents include hypotension.

____ 7. The precise action of hormones on malignant neoplasms is unknown.

____ 8. Gonadal hormones are used in carcinomas of the reproductive tract and advanced breast cancer.

____ 9. The most serious adverse effects of antitumor antibiotics are high blood cell counts and strokes.

____ 10. Alkylating agents are the newest group of antineoplastic agents.

ANSWER KEY

Multiple Choice

1. D	2. D	3. C	4. A	5. C
6. B	7. C	8. A	9. C	10. A
11. B	12. B	13. C	14. A	15. B
16. D	17. B	18. C	19. A	20. B

Matching—Terms and Descriptions

1. F	2. E	3. D	4. C	5. A	6. B

Matching—Drug Names

1. H	2. E	3. G	4. F	5. A
6. D	7. C	8. B		

Fill in the Blank

1. metastasize	2. *tumor*	3. many days
4. chemotherapy	5. curable	6. radiation
7. DNA	8. leukopenia	9. not known
10. leukemias	11. feminization	12. congestive heart
13. nitrogen mustard	14. ovarian	15. mitotic
16. mitosis (M)	17. purine	18. Methotrexate
19. hormone	20. Velban®	

True or False

1. F	2. F	3. F	4. T	5. T
6. F	7. T	8. T	9. F	10. F

CHAPTER 21

Analgesics

Multiple Choice

Select the correct answer from choices A–D.

1. Use of aspirin during viral infections in children is associated with an increased incidence of which of the following?

    A. coronary thrombosis
    B. blood clots in small arteries

    C. Reye syndrome
    D. osteoarthritis

2. Acetaminophen has little effect on which of the following?

    A. treating mild to moderate pain
    B. platelet adhesion

    C. fever
    D. none of the above

3. Which of the following agents is not a nonsteroidal anti-inflammatory drug (NSAID)?

    A. meclofenamate
    B. naltrexone

    C. indomethacin
    D. celecoxib

4. Which of the following is the newest COX-2 inhibitor?

    A. celecoxib
    B. rofecoxib

    C. meloxicam
    D. levorphanol

5. Which of the following is the major adverse effect of opioid analgesics?

    A. insomnia
    B. diarrhea

    C. pulmonary edema
    D. respiratory depression

6. Acute acetaminophen poisoning may produce all of the following, except:

    A. hyperglycemia
    B. hepatic coma

    C. acute renal failure
    D. leukopenia

7. Which of the following is the generic name for Oruvail®?

    A. ibuprofen
    B. fenoprofen

    C. ketoprofen
    D. etodolac

8. Common adverse effects of high doses of aspirin include:

    A. dyspepsia and epigastric pain
    B. diarrhea and constipation

    C. headache and a fever
    D. A and B

9. Which of the following agents are contraindicated in patients with chicken pox and influenza in children?

    A. morphine sulfate
    B. aspirin

    C. acetaminophen
    D. ampicillin

10. Most of the nonsteroidal anti-inflammatory drugs have:

    A. analgesic and antipyretic effects   C. anticoagulant effects
    B. antineoplastic effects   D. antibiotic effects

11. Which of the following substances is an enzyme?

    A. cortisol   C. prostaglandin
    B. COX-1 and COX-2   D. B and C

12. Which of the following cyclooxygenase inhibitors was removed from the U.S. market by the FDA?

    A. rofecoxib   C. meloxicam
    B. celecoxib   D. prostaglandin

13. A deformity of the spinal column causing a hunchbacked appearance is referred to as which of the following?

    A. osteoarthritis   C. kyphosis
    B. osteomyelitis   D. lordosis

14. Which of the following is the generic name for Clinoril®?

    A. piroxicam   C. nabumetone
    B. sulindac   D. tolmetin

15. COX-2 inhibitors are contraindicated in which of the following patients?

    A. those who have joint pain   C. those who have asthma
    B. those who have dysmenorrhea   D. those who have backache

16. Most of the currently used opioid analgesics are primarily located at the:

    A. delta receptors   C. kappa receptors
    B. mu receptors   D. gamma receptors

17. Which of the following is not an indication of narcotic analgesics?

    A. pulmonary edema   C. severe constipation
    B. persistent cough   D. myocardial infarction

18. Which of the following is the generic name for Darvon®?

    A. propoxyphene   C. levorphanol
    B. oxycodone   D. methadone

19. Which of the following is an opioid?

    A. naltrexone   C. oxaprozin
    B. meperidine   D. naproxen

20. Opioid antagonist drugs should be used with caution in which of the following?

    A. partial reversal of opioid effects   C. hypotension
    B. opioid overdosage   D. neonates and children

Matching—Terms and Descriptions

Match the lettered term to its numbered description.

Description

1. _____ They can combine with receptors to initiate drug actions

2. _____ A synthetic narcotic substance

3. _____ Increases vasodilation and contracts smooth muscle

4. _____ An unpleasant sensation with potential tissue damage

5. _____ An enzyme that is essential for the inflammation process

6. _____ Altering perception without producing anesthesia

Term

A. Bradykinin

B. Opioid

C. Analgesic

D. Cyclooxygenase

E. Opioid antagonists

F. Pain

Matching—Drug Names

Match the generic and trade names.

Generic Name

1. _____ thiosalicylate

2. _____ diflusinal

3. _____ ibuprofen

4. _____ diclofenac

5. _____ nalmefene

6. _____ ketoprofen

7. _____ choline salicylate

8. _____ acetaminophen

Trade Name

A. Oruvail®

B. Arthropan®

C. Tempra®

D. Revex®

E. Voltaren®

F. Dolobid®

G. Motrin®

H. Rexolate®

Fill in the Blank

Select terms from your reading to fill in the blanks.

1. Pure opioid antagonists such as naloxone are able to block both _____ and _____ receptors.

2. The mechanism of action of NSAIDs is _____.

3. Acetaminophen should not be used with _____.

4. Opioid antagonists are contraindicated in respiratory depression due to _____ drugs.

5. Anti-inflammatory effects of the nonsteroidal anti-inflammatory drugs may develop only after _____ of treatment.

6. Aspirin may be useful in the prevention of coronary _____ by prolonging bleeding time.

7. Indomethacin, piroxicam, and celecoxib are examples of _____.

8. Salicylates that are combined with caffeine can, in very large doses, cause _____ in a developing fetus.

9. Acetaminophen may be used as a substitute for _____ when the latter is not tolerated.

10. Intolerance is relatively common with aspirin and includes rash, _____, rhinitis, edema, or an anaphylactic reaction with _____.

11. In low doses, baby aspirin appears to affect blood clotting by inhibiting _____ formation.

12. Aspirin and ibuprofen are available as inexpensive _____ drugs.

13. New forms of ergotamine are available as _____ tablets, which provide a more readily _____ and rapid-acting treatment.

14. The drugs of choice for treatment of _____ are often the triptans.

15. Synthetic narcotics are produced in laboratories, with _____ properties.

16. Herbal supplements such as yohimbe may increase the effects of _____.

17. Most NSAIDs are used for _____ conditions such as arthritis, osteoarthritis, dysmenorrhea, and dental pain.

18. Intracranial headaches result from _____ inside the skull.

19. Narcotic analgesics are classified as _____ drugs, except for heroin, which is classified as a _____ drug.

20. The route of administration of naltrexone (ReVia®) is _____; and for naloxone (Narcan®), the route is _____.

True or False

Select the letter "T" or "F" for the following questions.

____ 1. The major adverse effects of triptans include: coronary artery vasospasm, heart attack, and cardiac arrest.

____ 2. Narcotic analgesics should be used cautiously in patients with toxic psychosis.

____ 3. Narcotic analgesics are used to manage severe constipation.

____ 4. COX-2 inhibitors should be used cautiously in patients with primary dysmenorrhea.

____ 5. Recently, meloxicam (Mobic®) was removed from the U.S. market due to problems that resulted in certain patients.

____ 6. Swelling of blood vessels is referred to as "angioedema."

____ 7. The FDA has approved celecoxib for the treatment of angina pectoris.

____ 8. Acetaminophen is safe in patients with hepatic disease.

____ 9. Aspirin may be useful in the prevention of stroke.

____ 10. Nonopioid analgesics are used for minor aches and pains.

ANSWER KEY

Multiple Choice

1. C	2. B	3. B	4. C	5. D
6. A	7. C	8. D	9. B	10. A
11. D	12. A	13. C	14. B	15. C
16. B	17. C	18. A	19. B	20. D

Matching—Terms and Descriptions

1. E	2. B	3. A	4. F	5. D	6. C

Matching—Drug Names

1. H	2. F	3. G	4. E	5. D
6. A	7. B	8. C		

Fill in the Blank

1. mu; kappa	2. unknown	3. alcohol
4. nonopioid	5. several weeks	6. thrombosis
7. NSAIDs	8. birth defects	9. aspirin
10. bronchospasm; shock	11. prostaglandin	12. OTC
13. sublingual; available	14. migraine	15. analgesic
16. morphine	17. inflammatory	18. increased pressure
19. Schedule II; Schedule I	20. oral; intravenous	

True or False

1. T	2. T	3. F	4. F	5. F
6. T	7. F	8. F	9. F	10. T

CHAPTER 22

Anti-Infectives and Systemic Antibacterial Agents

Multiple Choice

Select the correct answer from choices A–D.

1. Which of the following phrases describes the elements of an infectious process?

   A. surgical asepsis
   B. chain of infection
   C. antimicrobial
   D. none of the above

2. Which of the following is a true statement regarding Gram stains?

   A. They can identify specific types of bacteria.
   B. They are capable of determining types of protozoa.
   C. They can differentiate viruses from fungi.
   D. They are capable of determining types of rickettsia.

3. Which of the following infectious diseases is caused by pathogenic bacteria?

   A. malaria
   B. typhus
   C. gonorrhea
   D. genital herpes

4. Rocky Mountain spotted fever is caused by which of the following types of microorganisms?

   A. viruses
   B. rickettsia
   C. fungi
   D. bacteria

5. Nonpathogenic microorganisms within the body may be disrupted by administration of oral antibiotics, which causes:

   A. radioactivity
   B. suppuration
   C. supraventricular arrhythmia
   D. superinfection

6. Sulfonamides are bacteriostatic; they suppress bacterial growth by triggering a mechanism that blocks:

   A. biosynthesis of nucleic acid and lipids
   B. folic acid synthesis
   C. beta-lactamase enzymes
   D. bacterial protein synthesis

7. During isoniazid therapy, the patient should be given which of the following vitamin supplements to prevent neuritis?

   A. vitamin C
   B. vitamin A
   C. vitamin K
   D. vitamin B_6

8. Clindamycin is indicated in serious infections when less toxic alternatives are inappropriate. Therefore, which of the following bone disorders should be treated with these agents?

    A. osteomyelitis
    B. osteoporosis

    C. osteosarcoma
    D. osteomalacia

9. Which of the following is a serious adverse effect of macrolides?

    A. osteoporosis
    B. infertility

    C. blurred vision
    D. severe coughing

10. Which of the following is the mechanism of action of cephalosporins?

    A. They inhibit cell wall synthesis by binding to penicillin-binding proteins.
    B. They inhibit bacterial growth by blocking folic acid synthesis.

    C. They inhibit protein synthesis.
    D. They inhibit viral growth by blocking folic acid synthesis

11. Which of the following is/are the adverse effect(s) of carbenicillin and ticarcillin?

    A. hypokalemia
    B. hyperlipidemia

    C. hypercalcemia
    D. hyperkalemia

12. Which of the following is a true statement regarding the third-generation of cephalosporins?

    A. They are effective against most Gram-positive organisms and some Gram-negative organisms.
    B. They have broader Gram-negative activity and less Gram-positive activity than do second-generation agents.

    C. They have the same effects on Gram-positive and Gram-negative organisms.
    D. They have the greatest action against Gram-negative organisms among the four generations.

13. Which of the following is the serious adverse effect of aminoglycosides?

    A. severe hypertension
    B. skin rash

    C. urticaria
    D. nephrotoxicity

14. The combination of amoxicillin and clavulanate potassium is contraindicated in which of the following infections?

    A. infectious mononucleosis
    B. otitis media

    C. sinusitis
    D. pneumonia

15. Which of the following is the generic name for Keflex®?

    A. cefadroxil
    B. cephalexin

    C. cefaclor
    D. ceftriaxone

16. Which of the following antibiotics are contraindicated in patients with tendonitis or any tendon problem?

    A. tetracyclines
    B. macrolides

    C. aminoglycosides
    D. fluoroquinolones

17. Which of the following is not an aminoglycoside?

    A. gentamicin
    B. azithromycin

    C. kanamycin
    D. tobramycin

18. Which of the following antibiotics are the drug of choice for the treatment of *Mycoplasma pneumoniae* and pertussis?

    A. isoniazid and rifampin
    B. sulfonamides

    C. penicillins
    D. macrolides

19. Ethambutol should be avoided for children under the age of:

   A. 6 years
   B. 10 years
   C. 15 years
   D. 18 years

20. Tetracyclines should not be used in children younger than:

   A. 6 years
   B. 8 years
   C. 10 years
   D. 18 years

Matching—Terms and Descriptions

Match the lettered term to its numbered description.

Description

1. _____ Killing bacterial growth

2. _____ Suppressing bacterial growth by blocking folic acid synthesis

3. _____ Ultramicroscopic organisms that lack rigid cell walls

4. _____ Bacteria in a resistant stage that can withstand an unfavorable environment

5. _____ Intercellular parasites that need to be in living cells to reproduce

6. _____ A group of enzyme disorders that cause skin problems

Term

A. Porphyria

B. Mycoplasms

C. Rickettsia

D. Spore

E. Bacteriostatic

F. Bactericidal

Matching—Drug Names

Match the generic and trade names.

Generic Name

1. _____ cloxacillin

2. _____ penicillin G procaine

3. _____ carbenicillin

4. _____ cefepime

5. _____ cefmetazole

6. _____ cefoxitin

7. _____ cefdinir

8. _____ ceftriaxone

Trade Name

A. Omnicef®

B. Maxipime®

C. Zefazone®

D. Geocillin®

E. Rocephin®

F. Crysticillin®

G. Mefoxin®

H. Cloxapen®

Fill in the Blank

Select terms from your reading to fill in the blanks.

1. The kidneys eliminate all cephalosporins except _____.

2. Aminoglycosides are _____; they inhibit bacterial protein synthesis.

3. Neomycin is the most nephrotoxic _____, and streptomycin is the least nephrotoxic.

4. Erythromycin generally penetrates the cell walls of Gram-_____ bacteria more readily than the cell walls of Gram-_____ bacteria.

5. Tetracycline should not be used during infancy, because they cause permanent discoloration of _____ in children.

6. Chloramphenicol should be avoided in the treatment of _____ infections.

7. Topical applications of clindamycin are used in the treatment of _____.

8. Dapsone is the primary agent for the treatment of all forms of _____.

9. Spectinomycin is used clinically for only one purpose: namely, to treat or prevent acute _____ when the organism is resistant to penicillin.

10. Vancomycin is used for the treatment of osteomyelitis, staphylococcal pneumonia, and _____.

11. Antitubercular drugs include streptomycin, rifampin, ethambutol, pyrazinamide, rifabutin, and _____.

12. Isoniazid is the most widely prescribed _____ drug.

13. Viruses are organisms that can live only _____.

14. Gram-positive microorganisms stain _____ or purple.

15. Contact with contaminated animate hosts such as animal or insects is referred to as _____ transmission.

16. Bacteria are classified according to their shape, such as bacilli, spirilla, and _____.

17. Infection from rickettsia is spread through the bites of fleas, mites, _____, and _____.

18. Hematuria and _____ are two of the major adverse effects of sulfonamide agents.

19. Penicillin G is ten times more active than _____ against Gram-negative organisms.

20. Injection of penicillin may cause a patient to experience anaphylactic reaction within _____ minutes after administration.

True or False

Select the letter "T" or "F" for the following questions.

____ 1. Penicillinase-resistant penicillins prevent cell wall synthesis by binding to enzymes called "penicillin-binding proteins."

____ 2. Extended-spectrum penicillins are prescribed mainly to treat serious infections caused by Gram-negative organisms, such as sepsis.

____ 3. Tetracyclines are known as beta-lactam antibiotics.

____ 4. The cephalosporins are classified into two different "generations."

____ 5. The most common adverse effects of cephalosporins include nausea, vomiting, diarrhea, and nephrotoxicity.

____ 6. Neomycin is used for pre-operative bowel sterilization, hepatic coma, and in topical form for burns.

____ 7. Tetracyclines are narrow-spectrum agents that are effective against certain bacterial strains.

____ 8. The indications of fluoroquinolones are primarily for the treatment of urinary tract and lower respiratory infections.

____ 9. Chloramphenicol should be given cautiously to patients with impaired hepatic or renal function.

____ 10. Vancomycin (in higher doses) may cause ototoxicity and nephrotoxicity.

ANSWER KEY

Multiple Choice

1. B	2. A	3. C	4. B	5. D
6. B	7. D	8. A	9. D	10. A
11. A	12. B	13. D	14. A	15. B
16. D	17. B	18. D	19. A	20. B

Matching—Terms and Descriptions

1. F	2. E	3. B	4. D	5. C	6. A

Matching—Drug Names

1. H	2. F	3. D	4. B	5. C
6. G	7. A	8. E		

Fill in the Blank

1. cefoperazone	2. bactericidal	3. aminoglycosides
4. positive; negative	5. teeth	6. minor
7. acne	8. leprosy	9. gonorrhea
10. endocarditis	11. isoniazid	12. antitubercular
13. inside cells	14. blue	15. vector borne
16. cocci	17. ticks; lice	18. crystalluria
19. penicillin V	20. 30	

True or False

1. T	2. T	3. F	4. F	5. T
6. T	7. F	8. T	9. T	10. T

CHAPTER 23

Antiviral, Antifungal, and Antiprotozoal Agents

Multiple Choice

Select the correct answer from choices A–D.

1. Which of the following agents is an example of a nucleoside reverse transcriptase inhibitor?

   A. lamivudine (Epivir®)
   B. efavirenz (Sustiva®)
   C. nevirapine (Viramune®)
   D. enfuvirtide (Fuzeon®)

2. Lamivudine is used in combination with zidovudine to treat which of the following infections?

   A. chronic hepatitis B
   B. herpes simplex virus
   C. HIV infection
   D. A and C

3. Which of the following is an antifungal drug?

   A. famciclovir
   B. itraconazole
   C. metronidazole
   D. iodoquinol

4. Which of the following is one of the miscellaneous agents for the treatment of HIV-AIDS?

   A. tenofovir
   B. acyclovir
   C. famciclovir
   D. ribavirin

5. Fungal infections include:

   A. cryptococcosis
   B. trichomoniasis
   C. histoplasmosis
   D. A and C

6. Metronidazole (Flagyl®) is the drug of choice in which of the following?

   A. mycoses
   B. giardiasis
   C. tinea
   D. *Candida* infections

7. Which of the following is not an amebicide?

   A. paromomycin (Humatin®)
   B. iodoquinol (Yodoxin®)
   C. nevirapine (Viramune®)
   D. doxycycline (Vibramycin®)

8. "Shingles" is also referred to as which of the following?

   A. varicella
   B. cytomegalovirus
   C. varicella-zoster
   D. anthrax

9. Oral acyclovir is indicated for the treatment of primary and recurrent:

   A. genital herpes
   B. herpes simplex encephalitis

   C. acute herpes zoster
   D. hepatitis C

10. The human body is generally resistant to infection by which of the following microorganisms?

    A. viruses
    B. fungi

    C. bacteria
    D. protozoa

11. Amphotericin B is used intravenously for all of the following fatal systemic fungal infections, except:

    A. blastomycosis
    B. coccidiomycosis

    C. aspergillosis
    D. *Candida albicans*

12. Vaginal tablets of nystatin are contraindicated in which of the following conditions?

    A. pregnancy
    B. trichomonal vaginitis

    C. *Candida albicans*
    D. A and B

13. All of the following disorders may be caused by protozoa, except:

    A. toxoplasmosis
    B. giardiasis

    C. histoplasmosis
    D. trypanosomiasis

14. Griseofulvin is fungistatic and deposited in which of the following body organs?

    A. kidneys
    B. skin

    C. liver
    D. bone

15. All of the following agents are HIV antivirals, except:

    A. stavudine (Zerit®)
    B. indinavir (Crixivan®)

    C. acyclovir (Zovirax®)
    D. abacavir (Ziagen®)

16. Ganciclovir is prescribed for which of the following?

    A. cytomegalovirus retinitis and transplant patients
    B. influenza A

    C. herpes zoster
    D. recurrent genital herpes

17. The incidence and mortality of AIDS has declined substantially since 1996 due to which of the following?

    A. educated patients and good personal hygiene
    B. lower transmission of AIDS via heterosexual people

    C. higher living standards of people
    D. highly active anti-retroviral therapy

18. Ritonavir is an anti-HIV drug that is classified as which of the following?

    A. a Non-Nucleoside Reverse Transcriptase Inhibitor (NNRTI)
    B. a Nucleoside Reverse Transcriptase Inhibitor (NRTI)

    C. a Protease Inhibitor (PI)
    D. a miscellaneous drug

19. Fluconazole is an antifungal that is used for which of the following infections?

    A. systemic mycoses
    B. superficial mycoses

    C. both systemic and superficial mycoses
    D. none of the above

20. Which of the following medications may cause a bitter taste in the mouth and vaginal dryness?

    A. metronidazole (Flagyl®)
    B. atovaquone (Mepron®)

    C. pyrimethamine (Daraprim®)
    D. paromomycin (Humatin®)

Matching—Terms and Descriptions

Match the lettered term to its numbered description.

Description	Term
1. _____ Fungal diseases	A. Epidemic
2. _____ Caused by the bite of an anopheles mosquito	B. Protozoa
3. _____ Intracellular parasites	C. Replication
4. _____ Single-celled parasites	D. Mycoses
5. _____ The process of reproduction	E. Malaria
6. _____ An outbreak of a disease	F. Viruses

Matching—Drug Names

Match the generic and trade names.

Generic Name	Trade Name
1. _____ enfuvirtide	A. Zerit®
2. _____ zidovudine	B. Hivid®
3. _____ didanosine	C. Symmetrel®
4. _____ zalcitabine	D. Vistide®
5. _____ acyclovir	E. Retrovir®
6. _____ cidofovir	F. Videx®
7. _____ amantadine	G. Zovirax®
8. _____ stavudine	H. Fuzeon®

Fill in the Blank

Select terms from your reading to fill in the blanks.

1. *Trichomona vaginalis* is usually transmitted through _____ contact.

2. The most important human parasite among the sporozoa is *Plasmodium*, which causes _____.

3. The mechanism of action of primaquine and quinine is _____.

4. Nystatin can temporarily affect the sense of taste, and thus decrease _____.

5. Griseofulvin must be avoided in patients with known hypersensitivity and severe _____ disease.

6. Amphotericin B is the most effective agent available for the treatment of most _____ fungal infections.

7. Metronidazole should be cautiously used in patients with coexistent candidiasis, alcoholism, and _____ disease.

8. It is important to begin treatment during the _____ stage in order to delay acute symptoms and the onset of full-blown AIDS.

9. One of the more serious effects of ritonavir is potentially fatal _____.

10. Itraconazole is an antifungal indicated in the treatment of histoplasmosis, aspergillosis, and _____.

11. Amphotericin B is used cautiously in patients with severe _____ depression or _____ function impairment.

12. There are four different types of *Plasmodium*: *P. falciparum*, *P. malariae*, _____, and _____.

13. Viruses are extremely small, and contain their _____ information in either DNA or RNA.

14. Acyclovir is most effective against HSV-1 and _____.

15. We now know that HIV kills _____.

16. Missing a single dose of HAART medication even twice a week can cause the development of _____ HIV.

17. Systemic mycoses more commonly affect the lungs, digestive organs, and _____.

18. The generic name for Fungizone® is _____.

19. Fluconazole has been shown to be effective against _____, as well as oropharyngeal and systemic candidiasis, both of which are commonly seen in _____ patients.

20. Tenofovir is used in combination with other antiretrovirals for the treatment of _____.

True or False

Select the letter "T" or "F" for the following questions.

____ 1. Most protozoa obtain their food from dead or decaying organic matter.

____ 2. Griseofulvin is antiviral, and is the drug of choice in varicella (chickenpox).

____ 3. Amantadine is also used for candidal diaper rashes.

____ 4. Econazole nitrate is also used for angina pectoris.

____ 5. Metronidazole is the drug of choice in malarial parasites.

____ 6. Nystatin is fungicidal and fungistatic.

____ 7. Varicella-zoster is also called "shingles."

____ 8. Inflammation of the cornea of the eyes is referred to as "cataract."

____ 9. The mechanism of the antiviral activity of amantadine is unknown.

____ 10. Histoplasmosis and cryptococcosis are protozoal infections.

ANSWER KEY

Multiple Choice

1. A	2. D	3. B	4. A	5. D
6. B	7. C	8. C	9. A	10. B
11. D	12. D	13. C	14. B	15. C
16. A	17. D	18. C	19. C	20. A

Matching—Terms and Descriptions

1. D	2. E	3. F	4. B	5. C	6. A

Matching—Drug Names

1. H	2. E	3. F	4. B	5. G
6. D	7. C	8. A		

Fill in the Blank

1. sexual	2. malaria	3. unknown
4. appetite	5. liver	6. systemic
7. liver	8. latent	9. pancreatitis
10. blastomycosis	11. bone marrow; renal	12. *P. vivax; P. ovale*
13. genetic	14. HSV_2	15. lymphocytes
16. drug-resistant	17. brain	18. amphotericin B
19. meningitis; AIDS	20. HIV	

True or False

1. T	2. F	3. F	4. F	5. F
6. T	7. T	8. F	9. T	10. F

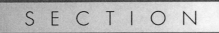

Pharmacology for Specific Populations

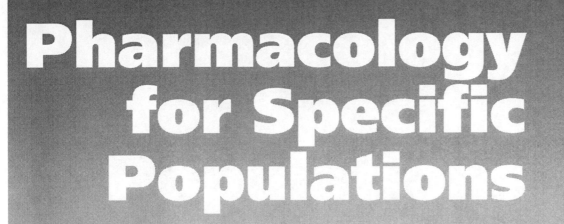

CHAPTER 24

Drug Therapy during Pregnancy and Lactation

Multiple Choice

Select the correct answer from choices A–D.

1. During pregnancy, to which of the following percentages does plasma volume increase?

   A. 15%
   B. 30%
   C. 50%
   D. 75%

2. Development of serious hypertension, along with fluid retention and loss of protein in the urine (that develops in pregnancy after the fifth month), is referred to as:

   A. malignant hypertension
   B. preeclampsia
   C. eclampsia
   D. kidney failure

3. Which of the following factors may affect drug metabolism?

   A. hepatic blood flow
   B. the diet (in general)
   C. liver disease
   D. all of the above

4. Methimazole is a common teratogenic drug that may be used as which of the following types of drugs?

   A. hormone replacement
   B. antithyroid
   C. antibiotic
   D. anticoagulant

5. It is believed by many experts that seizures in a pregnant woman can cause which of the following?

   A. brain damage
   B. hypoglycemia
   C. fetal hypoxia
   D. A and C

6. Which of the following is the treatment of choice for gestational diabetes after the baby is delivered?

   A. insulin therapy
   B. oral hypoglycemic drugs
   C. A and B
   D. none of the above

7. Which of the following agents is the best to treat hyperemesis gravidarum?

   A. piperazines
   B. phenothiazines
   C. phenobarbital
   D. vitamin B_{12}

8. Which of the following adverse effects occur because of cigarette smoking during pregnancy?

   A. withdrawal
   B. renal failure
   C. premature birth and intrauterine growth retardation
   D. neonatal depression

9. Which of the following adverse effects occurs because of taking acetaminophen during pregnancy?

   A. neonatal depression   C. premature birth
   B. renal failure   D. intrauterine growth retardation

10. Women with diabetes are at risk for having babies with:

    A. hypocalcemia   C. higher birth weight
    B. hypertension   D. all of the above

11. Which of the following adverse effects occurs because of using cocaine during pregnancy?

    A. vascular disruption, withdrawal, and intrauterine   C. electrolyte imbalance
       growth retardation   D. renal failure
    B. adrenocortical suppression

12. The actions and properties of drugs are referred to as:

    A. pharmacokinetics   C. pharmacopoeia
    B. pharmacognosy   D. pharmacodynamics

13. Controlled studies in pregnant women show that there is no risk to the fetus when a drug is used from:

    A. category A   C. category C
    B. category B   D. category D

14. During the period of organogenesis, teratogenic drugs may cause serious:

    A. malnutrition   C. malformations
    B. melanomas   D. malaise

15. Women should not breastfeed while they are taking:

    A. folic acid   C. active radioactive agents
    B. penicillin   D. fish oil

16. The drug of choice for preeclampsia, to prevent convulsions, is which of the following agents?

    A. hydralazine   C. furosemide
    B. magnesium sulfate   D. mannitol

17. Which of the following antibiotics are listed as common teratogenic drugs?

    A. tetracyclines   C. cephalosporins
    B. penicillins   D. aminoglycosides

18. High doses of fluoxetine (Prozac®) during pregnancy have been shown to cause:

    A. higher birth weight   C. lower blood sugar
    B. lower birth weight   D. higher blood sugar

19. Which of the following is the most serious condition during pregnancy?

    A. depression   C. malnutrition
    B. iron deficiency anemia   D. eclampsia

20. Drugs can be distributed in a mother's breast milk, usually in:

    A. high concentrations   C. low calories
    B. low concentrations   D. high calories

Matching—Teratogenic Drugs

Match the lettered indication to the numbered drug or drug class.

Drug or Drug Class	Indications
1. _____ phenytoin	A. Psoriasis
2. _____ lithium	B. Anticoagulant
3. _____ isotretinoin	C. Antineoplastic
4. _____ coumarin	D. Antimanic
5. _____ busulfan	E. Acne
6. _____ etretinate	F. Anticonvulsant

Fill in the Blank

Select terms from your reading to fill in the blanks.

1. By the 32nd week of pregnancy, a woman's cardiac output has increased by _____ percent.

2. Pregnancy drug categories were developed in 1980 by the _____ to help classify drugs according to the risks they pose to a developing fetus.

3. Many of the side effects of pregnancy can mask the _____ of drug therapy in pregnant patients.

4. The use of benzodiazepines can cause _____ infant syndrome.

5. The American Academy of Pediatrics published a report in 2001 that identified several _____ of drugs that may cause problems during breastfeeding.

6. Drugs such as selective serotonin reuptake inhibitors (SSRIs) do not appear to cause _____ risk for fetal complications.

7. Gestational diabetes may develop in _____ percent of all pregnancies and resolves after birth.

8. Preeclampsia is characterized by _____, cerebral edema, and proteinuria.

9. Fat-soluble substances are referred to as _____.

10. Floppy infant syndrome is also called infantile _____.

11. The heart rate in a pregnant woman increases by about _____ beats per minute.

12. The fetus receives drugs from the mother's circulatory system, which _____ drugs through the _____.

13. In some patients, preeclampsia may progress to _____.

14. The embryonic phase is completed at about _____ days, when the fetal phase begins.

15. Drugs are affected by pregnancy _____, which can result in a larger than normal amount of free drugs in circulation.

16. The use of _____ is preferred over _____ drugs for women who have developed gestational diabetes.

17. Antiemetic drugs that are used for pernicious vomiting during pregnancy include _____ and phenothiazines.

18. Eclampsia is a serious condition that may cause _____ seizures.

19. The actions of blood in the body are referred to as _____.

20. The actions and properties of drugs are known as _____.

True or False

Select the letter "T" or "F" for the following questions.

_____ 1. Pregnancy drug categories are divided into five subgroups.

_____ 2. Animal studies do not always accurately predict human responses to the studied drug.

_____ 3. The force that impels certain atoms to unite with certain other atoms is referred to as "teratogenicity."

_____ 4. Agents that cause the development of gestational diabetes are called "teratogenic."

_____ 5. Low blood pressure, weight loss, and glucose in the urine represent preeclampsia.

_____ 6. The blood volume increases by 40 percent during pregnancy.

_____ 7. The mechanism of action of any drug that is used in pregnant women has important clinical applications.

_____ 8. Adverse fetal effects of high doses of phenobarbital include neonatal depression and premature birth.

_____ 9. Anticonvulsant drug therapy may adversely affect a developing fetus.

_____ 10. Valproic acid should be avoided in pregnant women.

ANSWER KEY

Multiple Choice

1. C	2. B	3. D	4. B	5. D
6. D	7. A	8. C	9. B	10. C
11. A	12. D	13. A	14. C	15. C
16. B	17. A	18. B	19. D	20. B

Matching—Teratogenic Drugs

1. F	2. D	3. E	4. B	5. C	6. A

Fill in the Blank

1. 50	2. FDA	3. adverse effects
4. floppy	5. categories	6. increased
7. 2 to 5	8. hypertension	9. lipophilic
10. hypotonia	11. 10 to 15	12. passes; placenta
13. eclampsia	14. 60	15. hormones
16. insulin, oral hypoglycemic	17. piperazines	18. generalized
19. hemodynamics	20. pharmacodynamics	

True or False

1. T	2. T	3. F	4. F	5. F
6. T	7. T	8. F	9. T	10. T

CHAPTER 25

Drug Therapy for Pediatric Patients

Multiple Choice

Select the correct answer from choices A–D.

1. Which of the following is the reason that topical medications are absorbed more rapidly by infants and children?

   A. They have a lesser ratio of body surface area to weight.
   B. They have a greater ratio of body surface area to weight.
   C. They have a lesser ratio of height to body surface area.
   D. They have a greater ratio of height to body surface area.

2. Which of the following describes the gastric pH of newborns?

   A. It is more alkaline.
   B. It is more acidic.
   C. It is almost neutral.
   D. none of the above

3. Which of the following is the percentage of body water in premature neonates?

   A. 50%
   B. 60%
   C. 65%
   D. 85%

4. Which of the following statements is true regarding children under two years of age and their immature blood-brain barrier?

   A. They have a decreased risk of CNS toxicity.
   B. They have a decreased risk of renal toxicity.
   C. They have an increased risk of CNS toxicity.
   D. They have an increased risk of renal toxicity.

5. Renal function increases rapidly during infancy, reaching adult levels by:

   A. 2 to 4 months of age
   B. 4 to 6 months of age
   C. 6 to 12 months of age
   D. 2 to 4 years of age

6. Which of the following is widely used in infants as an antipyretic?

   A. ibuprofen
   B. aspirin
   C. acetaminophen
   D. both A and C

7. All of the following classes of drugs are used for asthma, except:

   A. bronchodilators
   B. glycosides
   C. leukotriene inhibitors
   D. corticosteroids

8. Which of the following microorganisms may cause epiglottitis in infants?

   A. *Haemophilus influenzae* type A
   B. *Haemophilus influenzae* type B
   C. *Pneumococci*
   D. *E. coli*

9. The incidence of croup is higher in:

   A. the late winter and early spring
   B. the late spring and early summer
   C. the late summer and early fall
   D. the late fall and early winter

10. The surgical procedure of inserting pressure-equalizing tubes into the tympanic membranes is referred to as a:

    A. myringotomy
    B. mastoidotomy
    C. myringoplasty
    D. stapedectomy

11. Which of the following is one of the most common congenital cardiovascular anomalies associated with maternal rubella (German measles) during early pregnancy?

    A. transposition of the great arteries
    B. patent ductus arteriosus
    C. atrial septal defect
    D. none of the above

12. Children with sickle cell anemia have abnormal:

    A. red blood cells
    B. white blood cells
    C. hemoglobin
    D. hematocrit

13. The peak age of onset for croup is:

    A. 6 months
    B. 12 months
    C. 18 months
    D. 24 months

14. Which of the following may be used to treat septicemia?

    A. oxacillin
    B. chloramphenicol
    C. ampicillin
    D. all of the above

15. Mortality and morbidity of acute bacterial meningitis in pediatric patients is:

    A. rare
    B. moderate
    C. significant
    D. only seen in tropical countries

Matching—Generic and Trade Names

Match the generic and trade names.

Generic Name	Trade Name
1. _____ zafirlukast	A. Flovent®
2. _____ theophylline	B. Rhinocort®
3. _____ salmeterol	C. Decadron®
4. _____ budesonide	D. Ventolin®
5. _____ cromolyn sodium	E. Serevent®
6. _____ albuterol	F. Intal®
7. _____ dexamethasone	G. Elixophyllin®
8. _____ fluticasone	H. Accolate®

Fill in the Blank

Select terms from your reading to fill in the blanks.

1. Approximately 80 percent of children with asthma have _____.

2. Respiratory distress syndrome is the result of the absence, deficiency, or alteration of the components of pulmonary surfactant. This syndrome is also called _____ disease.

3. Pneumonia in children is caused by viruses, bacteria, _____ organisms, and aspiration of foreign substances.

4. Bacteremia associated with active disease, whether localized or systemic, is referred to as _____.

5. The time from birth to approximately four weeks of age is called the _____ period.

6. In newborns, gastric pH is more _____, becoming more _____ at around 2 to 3 years of age.

7. Pharmacokinetics focuses on how drugs _____ throughout the _____.

8. Two factors that influence oral drug absorption are gastric emptying time and _____.

9. A condition characterized by blue coloring of the skin and mucous membranes is called _____.

10. The kidneys of infants younger than _____ months of age are not very well developed.

11. The inflammation of the tissue above the tongue in the airway is referred to as _____.

12. The administration of inhibitors of prostaglandin synthesis, such as indomethacin, is indicated in newborns for the treatment of _____.

13. The most common infectious agents causing bacterial meningitis in _____ include *Haemophilus influenzae* type B and *Streptococcus pneumoniae*.

14. Group A _____ are the most common bacteria causing acute pharyngitis.

15. Hepatic enzyme activity is not mature until _____ to _____ years of age.

16. Sickle cell traits occur in _____ percent of African Americans.

17. _____ is the drug of choice for the treatment of streptococcal infections.

18. Initial therapy in the treatment of bacterial meningitis includes immediate administration of _____ antibiotics.

19. Lipid-soluble drugs can be stored in body _____ as they have a high affinity for adipose tissue.

20. An inflammation of the lungs impairing breathing is called _____.

True or False

Select the letter "T" or "F" for the following questions.

____ 1. Neonates, infants, and young children have less body water than adults.

____ 2. Body fat percentage peaks at about 9 months of age and decreases between 1 and 5 years of age.

____ 3. Young children have lower metabolic rates and metabolize drugs more rapidly.

____ 4. During infancy, reduced renal excretion causes shorter drug half-lives and the increased possibility of toxicity to drugs primarily excreted through the renal system.

____ 5. Iron deficiency anemia is generally not evident until nine months of age.

____ 6. Diarrhea is one of the least common problems encountered by pediatricians.

___ 7. Leukotriene inhibitors include aminophylline and cromolyn sodium.

___ 8. Budesonide and fluticasone are classified as mast cell stabilizers.

___ 9. Children six years of age and younger are at particular risk for otitis media.

___ 10. Type I diabetes usually starts with polyphagia, weight loss, polydipsia, and polyuria.

ANSWER KEY

Multiple Choice

1. B	2. A	3. D	4. C	5. C
6. D	7. B	8. B	9. D	10. A
11. B	12. C	13. D	14. D	15. C

Matching—Generic and Trade Name

1. H	2. G	3. E	4. B	5. F
6. D	7. C	8. A		

Fill in the Blank

1. allergies	2. hyaline membrane	3. Mycoplasma
4. septicemia	5. neonatal	6. alkaline; acidic
7. move; body	8. pH	9. cyanosis
10. six	11. epiglottitis	12. patent ductus arteriosus
13. infants	14. streptococci	15. 1; 2
16. 8 to 10	17. Penicillin	18. multiple
19. fat	20. pneumonitis	

True or False

1. F	2. T	3. F	4. F	5. T
6. F	7. F	8. F	9. T	10. T

Drug Therapy in Geriatrics

Multiple Choice

Select the correct answer from choices A–D.

1. In the lymphatic system, age-related changes affect:

   A. nervous response
   B. immune responses

   C. drug metabolism
   D. drug absorption

2. Which of the following is the second leading cause of blindness in the world?

   A. iron deficiency anemia
   B. vitamin A deficiency

   C. glaucoma
   D. cataracts

3. Osteoporosis can develop insidiously with increasing deformity, known as:

   A. kyphosis
   B. lordosis

   C. scoliosis
   D. rickets

4. To prevent drug toxicity, which of the following organ's functions must be estimated, with the dosage of the drug adjusted accordingly?

   A. lungs
   B. kidneys

   C. bones
   D. stomach and pancreas

5. Trimethobenzamide hydrochloride (Tigan®) is classified as a:

   A. decongestant
   B. antihypertensive

   C. antiemetic
   D. antipsychotic

6. Thiazides (diuretics) can, in elderly patients, potentially worsen which of the following conditions?

   A. gout
   B. hypertension

   C. hypoglycemia
   D. renal failure

7. Which of the following is an important goal in chronic atrial fibrillation?

   A. prevention of possible thromboembolism
   B. prevention of stroke

   C. prevention of hepatic failure
   D. inhibition of cardiac arrest

8. More than 60 percent of hearts at ages 55 to 64 years show vascular:

   A. spasm
   B. clot

   C. dilation
   D. calcification

9. In postmenopausal women, reduction of which of the following hormones has been linked to increased incidences of osteoporosis and cardiovascular disease?

A. prolactin

B. estrogen

C. oxytocin

D. cortisol

10. Which of the following statements is not true regarding the gastrointestinal system and age-related changes?

A. Oral disorders are common among the elderly.

B. Gastric secretion declines with age.

C. Gastric cell function increases and gastric pH decreases.

D. Gastric emptying is reduced by stress, lack of ambulation, and diabetes mellitus.

11. Which of the following is the second-most common problem of the ears of elderly patients?

A. otitis media

B. hearing impairment

C. deafness

D. ear wax

12. Which of the following is not true regarding physiological changes due to aging?

A. Motor nerves deteriorate and slow reaction time.

B. The heart becomes less efficient.

C. Muscles of the bladder weaken, causing loss of urine control.

D. Tear production increases and nails grow more rapidly.

13. Which of the following is the most significant unchangeable risk factor for stroke?

A. elevated blood cholesterol

B. advanced age

C. advanced heart failure

D. elevated hypertension

14. Which of the following is the most common chronic ailment in elderly persons?

A. osteoporosis

B. dry eye syndrome

C. arthritis

D. renal failure

15. Polypharmacy is more common in which of the following groups?

A. elderly patients

B. pregnant women

C. newborn babies

D. teenagers

Matching—Drugs and Their Classifications

Match the letter of the drug that corresponds with its numbered classification.

Classification	Drug
1. _____ muscle relaxant	A. Phenergan®
2. _____ decongestant	B. Aldomet®
3. _____ antispasmodic	C. Talwin®
4. _____ antihistamine	D. Indocin®
5. _____ sedative-hypnotic	E. Bentyl®
6. _____ NSAID	F. Xanax®
7. _____ analgesic	G. Sudafed®
8. _____ antihypertensive	H. Soma®

Fill in the Blank

Select terms from your reading to fill in the blanks.

1. Alzheimer's disease is characterized by progressive _____ and cognitive function impairment.

2. Drug doses should be decreased if the patient has decreased renal drug _____, or the drug has a prolonged _____.

3. _____ are a leading cause of blindness and visual impairment worldwide.

4. Osteoarthritis is characterized by degeneration of _____, bone remodeling, and overgrowth of _____.

5. The major causes of death and morbidity associated with hypertension are myocardial infarction and _____.

6. Due to aging, metabolism slows down and causes weight _____.

7. The amount of collagen and elastin in the _____ decreases as people age, accounting for the _____ and wrinkling of the skin in elderly persons.

8. _____ replacement may be the treatment of choice in patients with severe osteoarthritis that cannot be adequately managed with other modalities.

9. Renal function declines progressively starting in the _____ decade, so that by age 70 normal renal function greatly declines in comparison with people at age 30.

10. A strong fibrous protein found in connective tissue is known as _____.

11. Aging alters pharmacodynamics and pharmacokinetics, affecting the choice, _____, and _____ of administration of many drugs.

12. Drug metabolism is often impaired in the elderly because of a decrease in the glomerular _____ rate, as well as reduced hepatic _____.

13. Antihypertensive drugs and influenza vaccines may benefit elderly persons by preventing or decreasing _____.

14. Common infections in the elderly include pneumonia, influenza, _____, and _____.

15. Glomerular filtration rate in elderly persons _____ by about 1 mL/min/year.

True or False

Select the letter "T" or "F" for the following questions.

____ 1. The peripheral glucose disposal rate is significantly lower in older than in younger persons.

____ 2. The skeletal systems of elderly people are affected by a decrease in total body mass.

____ 3. Lung weight with age increases dramatically, and chest wall compliance also increases.

____ 4. As many as 90 percent of older people experience traumatic lesions of the oral cavity, which may be ulcerative, atrophic, or hyperplasic.

____ 5. The reduction in hepatic clearance is due to the increased activity of microsomal enzymes and reduced hepatic perfusion with aging.

____ 6. Bleeding is a fairly common complication from ulcers in elderly persons.

____ 7. Constipation is common in elderly people because of alteration of motility in the stomach.

_____ 8. Serotonin (a neurotransmitter) is implicated in a variety of neural functions, such as pain, appetite, sleep, and sexual behavior.

_____ 9. As men age, testosterone levels increase, sperm production slows, and the testicles increase in size and firmness.

_____ 10. Aspirin has been shown to significantly reduce mortality, reinfarction, and stroke rate after acute myocardial infarction in older patients.

ANSWER KEY

Multiple Choice

1. B	2. C	3. A	4. B	5. C
6. A	7. A	8. D	9. B	10. C
11. B	12. D	13. B	14. C	15. A

Matching—Drugs and Their Classifications

1. H	2. G	3. E	4. A	5. F
6. D	7. C	8. B		

Fill in the Blank

1. memory	2. clearance; half-life	3. Cataracts
4. cartilage; bone	5. stroke	6. gain
7. dermis; thinning	8. Joint	9. fifth
10. collagen	11. dose; rate	12. filtration; clearance
13. morbidity	14. urinary tract; herpes zoster (shingles)	15. declines

True or False

1. T	2. T	3. F	4. F	5. F
6. T	7. F	8. T	9. F	10. T

CPSIA information can be obtained
at www.ICGtesting.com
Printed in the USA
FFOW01n1509030815
15695FF